Eagan Press Handbook Series

High-Fiber Ingredients

Amy L. Nelson

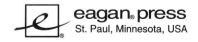

eagan press
St. Paul, Minnesota, USA

Cover: Fig powder courtesy of Valley Fig Growers;
prune/plum courtesy of the California Prune Board;
fluorescence micrograph image of dietary fiber from cereal grain
courtesy of Gary Fulcher, University of Minnesota, Department of Food
Science and Nutrition.

Library of Congress Catalog Card Number: 2001086118
International Standard Book Number: 1-891127-23-3

Printed in the United States of America on acid-free paper

American Association of Cereal Chemists
3340 Pilot Knob Road
St. Paul, Minnesota 55121-2097, USA

About the Eagan Press Handbook Series

The Eagan Press Handbook series was developed for food industry practitioners. It offers a practical approach to understanding the basics of food ingredients, applications, and processes—whether the reader is a research chemist wanting practical information compiled in a single source or a purchasing agent trying to understand product specifications. The handbook series is designed to reach a broad readership; the books are not limited to a single product category but rather serve professionals in all segments of the food processing industry and their allied suppliers.

In developing this series, Eagan Press recognized the need to fill the gap between the highly fragmented, theoretical, and often not readily available information in the scientific literature and the product-specific information available from suppliers. It enlisted experts in specific areas to contribute their expertise to the development and fruition of this series.

The content of the books has been prepared in a rigorous manner, including substantial peer review and editing, and is presented in a user friendly format with definitions of terms, examples, illustrations, and trouble-shooting tips. The result is a set of practical guides containing information useful to those involved in product development, production, testing, ingredient purchasing, engineering, and marketing aspects of the food industry.

Acknowledgment of Sponsors for *High-Fiber Ingredients*

Eagan Press would like to thank the following companies for their financial support of this handbook:

Cargill, Incorporated
Cedar Rapids, IA
319/399-2111

Nutrinova
Somerset, NJ
800/786-3883

Danisco Sweeteners
Ardsley, NY
914/674-6300

Opta Food Ingredients, Inc.
Bedford, MA
781/276-5100

Imperial Sensus, LLC
Sugar Land, TX
281/490-9522

J. Rettenmaier USA LP
Schoolcraft, MI
877/895-4099

International Fiber Corporation
North Tonawanda, NY
888/698-1963

TIC Gums, Inc.
Belcamp, MD
800/221-3953

Medallion Laboratories
Minneapolis, MN
763/764-4453

Eagan Press has designed this handbook series as practical guides serving the interests of the food industry as a whole rather than the individual interests of any single company. Nonetheless, corporate sponsorship has allowed these books to be more affordable for a wide audience.

Acknowledgments

Eagan Press thanks the following individuals for their contributions to the preparation of this book:

Mike Beavan, Watson Foods Co., Inc., West Haven, CT

Stuart Craig, Dansico Cultor, Ardsley, NY

Guy Crosby, Opta Food Ingredients, Inc., Bedford, MA

Jim Degen, California Prune Board, Pleasanton, CA

Jon DeVries, General Mills, Inc., Minneapolis, MN

Will Duensing, Bunge Lauhoff Grain Co., Danville, IL

Janet Gelroth, American Institute of Baking, Manhattan, KS

Jane Petrolino, Colloides Naturel, Inc., Bridgewater, NJ

Norm Greenburg, Novartis, Minneapolis, MN

Steve Haralampu, Opta Food Ingredients, Inc., Bedford, MA

Peter Hellstrom, Danisco Sugar/Fibrex, Malmö, Sweden

George Inglett, USDA-ARS, Peoria, IL

Julie Miller Jones, College of St. Catherine, St. Paul, MN

Gary Jue, Valley Fig Growers, Fresno, CA

Greg Kesel, Protein Technologies International, St. Louis, MO

Richard Lamb, Larex, Inc., Minneapolis, MN

Loren Larson, Opta Food Ingredients, Inc., Bedford, MA

Lars Lindhoff, Danisco Sugar/Fibrex, Malmö, Sweden

Larry Mckee, International Fiber Corp., North Tonawanda, NY

Kris Nelson, Grain Millers, Inc., Eden Prairie, MN

Ed Newton, The RiceX Co., El Dorado Hills, CA

Kathy Niness, Orafti Active Food Ingredients, Malvern, PA

Kaisa Poutanen, VTT Biotechnology and Food Research, Espoo, Finland

Ed Schmidt, Fiberich Technologies, Inc., St. Louis Park, MN

Scott Summers, Tree Top, Inc., Selah, WA

Bryan Tungland, Imperial Sensus, LLC, Sugar Land, TX

Dara Walter, The Pillsbury Co., Minneapolis, MN

Florian Ward, TIC Gums, Inc., Belcamp, MD

Fred White, National Starch and Chemical Co., Bridgewater, NJ

George Wornson, Barley's Best, Whitefish Bay, WI

Contents

Defining High-Fiber Ingredient Terminology

Fiber is an important aspect of diet and nutrition. It plays a role in many physiological digestive functions, such as providing bulk for waste elimination and regulating blood glucose and lipid levels. Traditionally, consumers have chosen foods such as whole grains, fruits, and vegetables as sources of dietary fiber. Recently, food manufacturers have responded to the consumer demand for foods with higher fiber content by developing products in which high-fiber ingredients are used. These ingredients have unique properties that raise the fiber level and also serve other functions in the formulation of food products. High-fiber ingredients can range from whole-meal flours of cereals to the exterior portion of shellfish. Synthetic ingredients such as polydextrose are also a source of high-fiber ingredients.

There are about 50 different types of high-fiber ingredients to choose from for developing a food product—a wide array of ingredients that encompasses a wide range of functionalities. Combining them with the ingredient processor's ability to tailor functions through processing leads to an even larger spectrum of choices. This handbook is written to help the food product developer and those involved in the manufacture of foods understand the properties, functions, and applications of high-fiber ingredients.

History of Dietary Fiber

Fiber is an important component in the structure of plants. Thus, it is often part of what we consume when we eat food materials made from plant sources. However, fiber as a dietary constituent has only recently been considered important. It is generally agreed that the term "dietary fiber" was first used in 1953 to describe the components of plant cell walls that were not digestible by humans (1). During the 1970s, scientists theorized that the high-fiber diets of Africans were responsible for their low incidence of diseases such as diabetes, heart disease, and colon cancer, which were common in Western countries (1). Since then, the term "dietary fiber" has been used to describe fibers consumed in foods that are important to human health, and the results of research on dietary fiber have filled volumes of texts, scientific journals, and other publications.

Research findings have led to further understanding of how fiber in plants and other materials is digested and how it influences human

Resistant starch—Starch resistant to enzyme attack in the human small intestine.

health, and methodologies have been developed to isolate components that are considered dietary fiber. The history of the development of the definition of dietary fiber and the analytical methodologies used to determine these components are reviewed elsewhere (1). Recently, the American Association of Cereal Chemists (AACC) developed an updated definition of dietary fiber to ensure that the term encompassed the complete characterization of the components of dietary fiber as well as their functions. The AACC, along with the Carbohydrate Technical Committee of the North American branch of the International Life Sciences Institute, was instrumental in developing the following definition:

> Dietary fiber is the edible parts of plants or analogous carbohydrates that are resistant to digestion and absorption in the human small intestine with complete or partial fermentation in the large intestine. Dietary fiber includes polysaccharides, oligosaccharides, lignin, and associated plant substances. Dietary fibers promote beneficial physiological effects including laxation, and/or blood cholesterol attenuation, and/or blood glucose attenuation.

This is a significant revision of the previously accepted fiber definition because it states that dietary fiber can be derived from sources other than plants. Polydextrose (a synthetically produced food ingredient) and chitin (an ingredient derived from shellfish) are materials that exhibit fiberlike physiological properties but are not derived from plants. The physiological function of dietary fiber is also included in the definition. This is significant because, as ingredients or components in foods are proven to affect physiological functions in the same way as dietary fiber, they may also be considered dietary fiber. Therefore, ingredients such as *resistant starch* may be considered sources of dietary fiber. Defining dietary fiber analytically is complex because the analytical methods that have been developed do not exactly replicate the human digestive system, which is part of the definition given above (2,3). Analytical methods for dietary fiber determination are discussed in detail in Chapter 2.

Composition

Dietary fibers include many components, which are often categorized by their solubility characteristics in the human digestive system. It is important to note the phrase "in the human digestive system." In other words, although a fiber may be called "soluble," it is not soluble in water in a molecular sense but forms a colloidal suspension in water. Soluble and insoluble fibers have different chemical characteristics and different physiological effects on the human body. Total dietary fiber (TDF) refers to the total amount of dietary fiber, both soluble and insoluble, in a food system.

INSOLUBLE DIETARY FIBERS

Insoluble dietary fibers are insoluble in aqueous solutions of enzymes that are designed to simulate the human digestive system. They are not digested in the human small intestine but may be fermented by bacteria in the large intestine. In general, these fibers increase bulk in the gastrointestinal tract and aid in waste elimination. Insoluble fibers include cellulose; hemicellulose; lignin; cutin, suberin, and other plant waxes; chitin and chitosan; and resistant starches.

Cellulose. Cellulose is the primary structural component of plant cell walls and is one of the most abundant organic compounds known. It is a linear, unbranched *polymer* of glucose units; thus, it is a *polysaccharide*. It is composed of the *monosaccharide* glucose in a β-D-1,4 glucosidic bond (Fig. 1-1). Native cellulose can have as many as 10,000–15,000 units per chain. The linear chains of cellulose can hydrogen-bond with each other to form very rigid, inflexible crystalline *microfibrils* up to 25 nm in diameter, or roughly a structure that is 30–100 chains wide (3). These structures give cellulose a strong, dense, partially crystalline, chemically and enzymatically resistant nature. Some cellulose (roughly 10%) can also exist in an *amorphous state.*

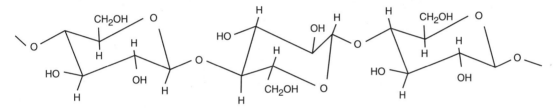

Fig. 1-1. Structure of cellulose, showing β-D-1,4 glucosidic bonds.

Cellulose is insoluble in hot or cold water and in dilute solutions of acids or bases. It has a high water-sorption capacity (see Chapter 2). Cellulose is resistant to degradation by human enzymes, but *cellulases* in microorganisms (which are present in the large intestine of humans) can attack the β-D-1,4 glucosidic bond.

Hemicellulose. The structures of hemicelluloses are more complex and varied than that of cellulose. In general terms, hemicelluloses are polysaccharides with several different monosaccharide units, which can singly, or in combination, make up the polymer backbone. They also may contain different types of side chain units, making hemicelluloses more difficult to define. Hemicelluloses have traditionally been described as insoluble in water and dilute solutions of acids but soluble in dilute solutions of bases. This definition distinguishes them from celluloses because celluloses are insoluble in dilute solutions of bases. Hemicelluloses are typically extracted from plant cell walls by using a base after pectin (a soluble fiber) is removed (3).

Hemicelluloses vary widely in structure. Their monosaccharide backbone units typically consist of β-1,4 glucosidic bonds of glucose, xylose, galactose, mannose, or arabinose, alone or in combination (Box 1-1). The hemicellulose polymers are often referred to by their monosaccharide component(s), using the *–an* suffix (e.g., xylan, arabinan, or glucomannan). Under this structural classification, all glucans could be considered hemicelluloses. However, the definition of

Polymer—A large molecule composed of monomer (i.e., single-unit) components.

Polysaccharide—A carbohydrate containing several hundred, thousand, or hundred thousand sugar units (from the Greek *poly*, meaning "many").

Monosaccharide—A carbohydrate containing one sugar unit, usually composed of five or six carbon atoms in a ring.

Microfibrils—Microscopic filamentous fibers.

Amorphous state—Having no crystalline state.

Cellulase—An enzyme that specifically cleaves glucose units from cellulose.

hemicelluloses is based on solubility, and β-glucans can differ in solubility depending on their polymer linkages. For example, a β-1,3 glucan (also called curdlan, discussed later in this chapter) is insoluble in water and dilute solutions of acids and is therefore a hemicellulose. The popular oat or barley β-glucan contains both β-1,3 and β-1,4 linkages and is water soluble, so it is not considered a hemicellulose. More discussion about soluble β-glucan is found later, in the soluble fiber section of this chapter.

The chain length of hemicellulose polymers can range from 50 to 200 monosaccharide units. Side chain units of the polymers can con-

Box 1.1. Typical Monosaccharides and Uronic Acids Found in Fibers

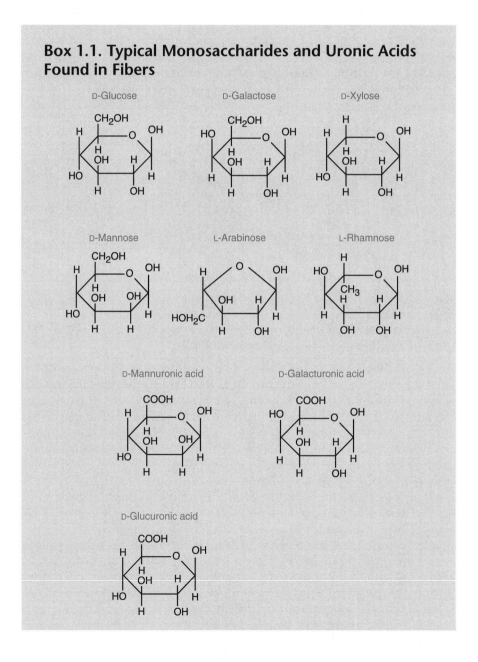

sist of uronic acids such as mannuronic, galacturonic, and glucuronic acids (Box 1-1). Pure hemicelluloses are typically not commercially available as high-fiber food ingredients because they can be difficult to isolate, which makes the processing more expensive.

Lignin. Lignin is not a polysaccharide. It is a polymer composed of the plant aromatic alcohols cinnamyl (e.g., *p*-coumaryl, confieryl, and sinapyl alcohols), syringyl, and guaicyl, which are also referred to as phenylpropane units. Thus, lignin is a polyphenylpropane polymer.

Lignin, which is highly insoluble in water, is responsible for the structural adhesion of the plant cell wall components because it excludes water when it forms networks by cross-linking with other saccharide-type molecules in plants. It is very resistant to chemical, enzymatic, and bacterial breakdown. Lignin is a very rigid component and is most associated with the structural integrity of wood. It can be selectively removed from certain high-fiber ingredients (e.g., oat hull fiber and wood pulp cellulose) during processing because of its high degree of insolubility. Lignin itself is not isolated as a commercially available high-fiber ingredient.

Cutin, suberin, and other plant waxes. Cutin and suberin are polyesters of hydroxy fatty acids. Other plant waxes consist of hydrocarbon chains. All are very insoluble in water. While they are by definition components of dietary fiber, they make up a small proportion of plant fibers and are not extracted for commercial use as high-fiber food ingredients.

Chitin and chitosan. Fungi, yeasts, and invertebrates have the ability to *polymerize* either of the amino sugars α-D-galactosamine or *N*-acetyl-α-D-glucosamine. The resultant polymer is called "chitin" and ranks second to cellulose as the most abundant polymer in nature (4). Chitin is very insoluble. Chitosan, a more soluble form of chitin, is produced by treating chitin with a strong base, which causes *deacylation*. Even though chitosan is soluble in dilute solutions of acid, both chitin and chitosan are considered insoluble fiber sources that can be used as high-fiber food ingredients.

Resistant starches. Starch is a polysaccharide found in granules in plant cells (Fig. 1-2). The starch granules contain two different polymeric forms of glucose, amylose and amylopectin. Amylose is a polymer of glucose in which the glucosidic bond is in the α-D-1,4 position. Amylopectin is a polymer of glucose with both α-D-1,4 and α-D-1,6 glucosidic bonds. The α-D-1,6 bond causes branching in the polymer chain. Plant starches are

Polymerize—Repeated linking of single units (monomers) of various chemical compounds, resulting in the creation of a polymer.

Deacylation—Removal of the acetyl group from a molecule. In the case of the chitosan polymer, this increases the solubility.

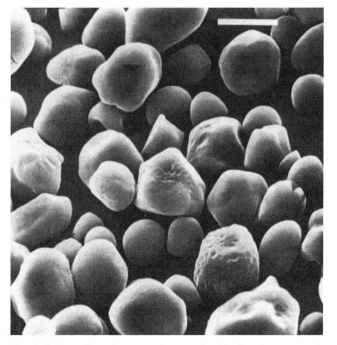

Fig. 1-2. Scanning electron micrograph of isolated corn starch granules. Bar = 10 µm. (Reprinted, with permission, from [5])

	Type of Resistant Starch	Occurrence
	RS1 - Physically inaccessible starch	Partially milled grains, seeds, and legumes
	RS2 - Granular starch	Banana starch, native potato starch
	RS3 - Nongranular, retrograded or crystalline starch	Ready-to-eat breakfast cereals, cooked and cooled potato
	RS4 - Chemically cross-linked starch	Produced through chemically cross-linking starch

Fig. 1-3. Schematic diagrams and definitions of resistant starch classes. (Adapted from [6]; courtesy of National Starch and Chemical Co.)

normally attacked by the amylase enzymes and are considered easily digested in the small intestine of humans.

Resistant starches are a class of starches that are not easily attacked by amylases in the small intestine. Like other fiber components such as cellulose, they undergo some degree of digestion in the large intestine. Their resistance to digestion in the small intestine qualifies this class of starches as dietary fiber.

There are four different types of resistant starches: RS1, RS2, RS3, and RS4 (Fig. 1-3). The RS1 starches are physically enclosed or entrapped in the plant system (for example, in a seed, partially milled grain, or legume) and are therefore resistant to enzyme degradation. In order to be digested, they must be freed by breaking the outer coating or seed coat of the enclosure.

RS2 starches are intact granules. Enzymes cannot easily attack them until they are *gelatinized*. Examples of resistant starches of the RS2 type are those found in uncooked peas, green bananas, and uncooked potatoes (6).

RS3 starches have been gelatinized and *retrograded* and are no longer in a granular form. They have been formed into a network via crystalline junction zones. Enzymes can attack gelatinized starches, but, because of the network produced by retrogradation, they cannot easily attack retrograded starches. RS3 starches are present in breads, cooked and cooled potatoes, ready-to-eat cereals that have been retrograded through processing, and as commercially available ingredients (6).

RS4 starches are chemically modified starches that contain cross-linking. These starches show some resistance to enzyme attack because access to the enzyme is restricted by the chemical cross-linking.

SOLUBLE DIETARY FIBERS

Soluble dietary fibers are soluble in aqueous solutions of enzymes that are typical of the human digestive system. Many soluble fibers can be precipitated in a solution of one part aqueous enzyme solution

Gelatinization—A process involving water and heat during which amylose and amylopectin become hydrated and the starch granule swells, leaching out the amylose and amylopectin.

Retrogradation—The process by which amylose and amylopectin polymers reassociate with each other and themselves.

and four parts ethanol. A number of soluble fibers have been shown to help lower blood cholesterol levels and regulate the body's use of glucose. Soluble fibers include pectins, β-glucan, gums, and inulin.

Pectins. Pectins are the largest source of soluble fiber in plant food materials. They are polymers of D-galacturonic acid (Box 1-1) with α-1,4 glucosidic bonds. The simple sugar rhamnose is also part of this backbone, and pectins are sometimes referred to as rhamnogalacturonans (2–4). Side chains consisting of galactose, glucose, rhamnose, and arabinose are also located on the polymer backbone. While they are generally water soluble, the overall solubility of pectins depends on the side chain constituents. These side chains are lost when pectins are commercially processed (4). The galacturonic acid backbone monomers can also be in a methyl ester form (Fig. 1-4). As the number of groups in the methyl ester form increases, the overall solubility decreases.

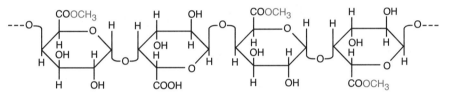

Fig. 1-4. Pectin molecule containing both acid groups and methyl ester (OCH$_3$) groups.

β-Glucan. The commonly known soluble fiber β-glucan is a polymer of glucose with mixed glucosidic bonds of both the β-1,3 and β-1,4 types. β-Glucans are often referred to as food gums or mucilage since they hydrate very well, forming viscous solutions. Grains are the primary source of β-glucans; barley and oats, in particular, contain high amounts of β-glucan. The β-glucan contents of several grains are shown in Table 1-1.

Gums. This category encompasses a large assortment of polymers that are water soluble. Different species of plants also contain different types and concentrations of gums. The polymers, in general, are composed of backbones and side chains of the monosaccharides and uronic acids listed in Box 1-1. Gums can also be produced by microbial fermentation (e.g., xanthan and gellan gum). Many gums are used at low levels in a food product because of their ability to affect functionality, such as building viscosity (e.g., guar and tragacanth gum). Some gums, however, can be used to increase the total dietary fiber content of a food product. The specific plant gums that are isolated for food ingredient use are listed in the section on production and processing below.

Inulin. Inulin is a linear polymer of fructose. It contains no side chains and no uronic acids groups and therefore is different from the

TABLE 1-1. β-Glucan Content of Selected Grains[a]

Grain	Percent
Barley	2.0–9.0
Oats	2.5–6.6
Rye	1.9–2.9
Wheat	0.5–1.5
Triticale	0.3–1.2
Sorghum	1.0
Rice	0.6
Maize	0.1

[a] Data from (2).

Degree of polymerization—
The molecular size of a polymer, e.g., the number of linked
units in a starch chain.

gums described above. Inulin occurs naturally in many plants. The
degree of polymerization of the inulin chain can vary; thus, different inulin polymers can have different functionalities. Like inulin, fructooligosaccharides (FOS) are linear polymers of fructose. They are typically defined as containing up to 10 fructose units. Therefore, FOS
can be considered a subcategory of inulins.

Production and Processing of High-Fiber Ingredients

Many high-fiber ingredients, with differing processing characteristics, are available for use in food products. The type of high-fiber ingredient used in the final product depends on many factors, for example, availability, cost, desired functionality (e.g., to increase the
dietary fiber content, to increase viscosity, or to be a fat mimetic), and
final product requirements. Many manufacturers of high-fiber ingredients can tailor their processing steps to meet their customers' unique
needs. The manufacturer or food formulator can also choose different
types of fiber from different sources, blending them to meet their
needs for one product. To better show all of the choices, high-fiber ingredients available for formulation of foods are listed below according to the source of the ingredient. These sources are cereals, plant extracts or isolates, fruits, and other sources.

CEREAL-BASED INGREDIENTS

Cereal grains are the most commonly known source for high-fiber
ingredients. Examples of these ingredients include wheat bran, oat
bran, and rye flour. A classic depiction of the cereal grain is shown in
Figure 1-5. The outermost layer of the grain is called
the hull. It protects the grain from the elements and is
typically composed of insoluble fibers. The bran layer,
the next inner layer of the hull, is composed of both
insoluble and soluble fibers. The germ is where the
lipids are most concentrated, but insoluble and soluble fibers are also located in the germ. The endosperm
is composed mainly of starch contained within the endosperm cells. Cell walls of the endosperm also contain soluble and insoluble fiber but to a lesser extent
than the hull and bran layers do. Different cereal grains
vary in their hull, bran, germ, and endosperm levels
and contents. These grains are discussed in more detail
later in this chapter.

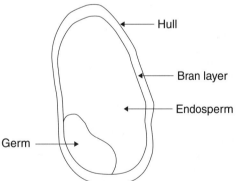

Fig. 1-5. Generalized structure of the cereal grain.

Generally, the milling of grains is a process designed
to separate the hull, bran, and germ from the starchy
endosperm (Fig. 1-6). Once the outer layers are separated from the endosperm, the components may go through all or some of the following steps: further separation (e.g., by *air classification*); grinding to a
specified granulation; bleaching to remove colors; stabilization to in-

Air classification—Separation
of components in a solid mixture by using air.

activate the enzymes that cause rancidity; defatting to remove lipids; and roasting or toasting to add colors and flavors. Various techniques of milling (as well as the type or cultivar of the grain itself) can produce various types of flours, brans, and germs. However, it is difficult to separate all three components during the milling process, so usually some proportion of each of the bran, germ, and starchy endosperm is present in any fraction.

Flours range from the whole-grain type, which contains most or all portions of the grain (e.g., whole wheat flour, about 11.8% TDF [4]) to flours that contain mainly the endosperm portion (e.g., all-purpose white flour, about 3.2% TDF [4]). Cereal brans are regarded as the most unrefined source of fiber. However, the concentrations of TDF in cereal brans are relatively low (Table 1-2). Corn bran, with a measured TDF of about 55%, is an exception to this rule.

High-fiber ingredients commonly come from grains such as oats, wheat, barley, rice, corn, rye; legumes (e.g., soybeans); and specialty grains such as amaranth. In general, because of their insoluble nature, cereal-based high-fiber ingredients are commonly used in the production of baked goods, cereals, and other extruded products such as snack items. When further modified (e.g., reduction of particle size to aid mouthfeel and/or suspension properties) or used in combination with other ingredients, cereal-based high-fiber ingredients can be used in applications such as beverages or dairy-based products. The processing steps of high-fiber ingredients derived from cereal grains are further detailed below.

Oats. Many products can be derived from oats, including rolled oats, steel cut oats, quick oats, baby oat flakes, instant oat flakes, oat flour, and oat bran, as well as other oat extracts. The more common high-fiber oat ingredients include oat fiber and oat bran, which are derived from the oat hulls and the oat bran/endosperm, respectively.

The oat hull covers the interior of the oat grain. The hull makes up about 25–30% by weight of the entire oat kernel (7,8). The fibers in the hull are typically composed of 50% hemicellulose, 30–40% cellulose, and 10–15% lignin. Oats are first cleaned, generally by screening or air classification, to remove foreign materials such as dust, chaff, weed seeds, and other grains. The hulls are then removed and can be further processed into high-fiber ingredients, which are commonly called

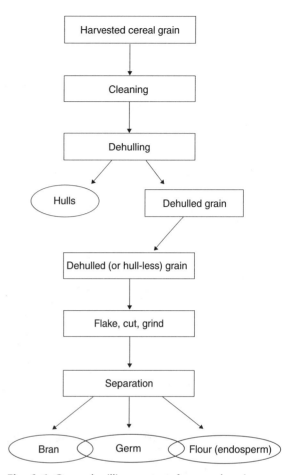

Fig. 1-6. General milling process for cereal grains.

TABLE 1-2. Total Dietary Fiber Contents of Cereal Brans

Bran Type	Total Dietary Fiber, %	Reference
Oat	16–32	(1,4)
Wheat	35–45	(4)
Barley	15–70	(4)
Rice	20–33	(7)
Corn	~55, 80–90	(4,10)
Soybean	~65	(4)
Rye	~25–30	(4)

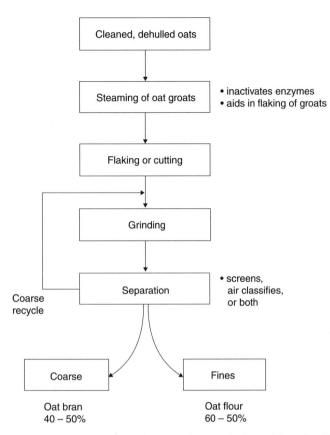

Cleaned, dehulled oats

Steaming of oat groats
• inactivates enzymes
• aids in flaking of groats

Flaking or cutting

Grinding

Separation
• screens,
  air classifies,
  or both

Coarse recycle

Coarse — Oat bran 40 – 50%

Fines — Oat flour 60 – 50%

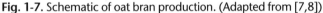

Fig. 1-7. Schematic of oat bran production. (Adapted from [7,8])

oat fibers. The hulls may be minimally processed (i.e., washed and ground) or given additional processing steps. Such steps may include an alkaline digestion process to remove lignin and increase the percentage of cellulosic materials, grinding to reduce particle size for improved mouthfeel, and/or bleaching to remove color. The TDF levels of oat fiber can vary depending on the process used but typically are about 90–98%, with about 80% of the oat fiber being present as cellulose.

The interior of the oat kernel, which is the bran layer, germ, and starchy endosperm, is commonly called the "groat." Oat bran is produced by separating the outer layer of the groat in a series of processing steps that generally include steaming, flaking, grinding, sifting, and air classification (Fig. 1-7). Oat bran is often stabilized to decrease rancidity. A thorough review of the processing details for the production of oat bran can be found elsewhere (7,8). With oats, it is particularly difficult to separate the bran layer from the starchy endosperm. Therefore, oat bran contains a high level of endosperm compared with wheat bran. However, β-glucan is highly concentrated in the cell walls of the endosperm, and thus oat bran is relatively high in β-glucan (7,8). The American Association of Cereal Chemists defined oat bran in 1989 (8) as

> . . . the food which is produced by grinding clean oat groats or rolled oats and separating the resultant oat flour by sieving, bolting, and/or other suitable means into fractions such that the oat bran fraction is not more than 50% of the starting material, and has a total β-glucan content of at least 5.5% (dry weight basis) and a total dietary fiber content of at least 16% (dry weight basis), and such that at least one-third of the total dietary fiber is soluble fiber.

This definition specifically states that the β-glucan content of oat bran must be at least 5.5%.

The TDF of oat brans available in the market can vary widely depending on how the manufacturer refines the product. The typical range is 16–32% TDF, with the proportion of soluble fiber being roughly equal to the insoluble fiber or at least one-third of the TDF (8,9). Oat brans with a TDF as high as 80–90% are also available, but these products have a lower β-glucan fraction because of the further separation of the endosperm from the bran during the refining process.

Other oat ingredients have been developed to meet the food industry's need for various functional ingredients. These ingredients have varying levels of TDF and derive much of their functionality from the presence of β-glucan. Fat mimetics derived from oat fiber starches and oat bran have been developed (9,10). The production of these types of ingredient involves the processing of oat flours and oat bran (e.g., enzymatic conversion of starches). β-Glucan levels can be tailored in these products from 1 to 15%. Aqueous extraction of whole oat groats has also led to the development of products that are used as sweetening agents. They can also provide functionality because of the presence of the soluble fiber β-glucan.

Wheat. The hull of the wheat kernel separates easily during threshing and is not used in the production of high-fiber ingredients. Wheat bran, wheat germs, and whole-wheat flours are commonly produced and used as high-fiber ingredients in foods. The type of wheat used to produce these ingredients can be either soft or hard wheat, red or white wheat, or durum wheat.

The milling of wheat is a very involved process, and an extensive review is found elsewhere (11). Simplified, the wheat kernel is cleaned and then *conditioned* to facilitate the removal of the bran from the endosperm. The kernel is then scoured to remove the bran. Defatting, inactivation of enzymes by heating, and/or grinding to reduce particle size can further refine the bran portion. The TDF of wheat brans can range from 35 to 90%, depending on the characteristics of the wheat used (i.e., hard or soft wheat) (9). Wheat brans can also differ depending on the wheat cultivar. Hard red wheat and hard white wheat differ in the genes for controlling bran color, but the overall brans can differ, too (10). The hard white wheat bran has a milder flavor and lighter color than the hard red wheat bran. Manufacturers of ready-to-eat cereals generally use either bran in their formulations, while manufacturers of bakery products tend to use brans from hard red wheat (10,12).

After the bran is removed, the wheat goes through a series of milling steps. The germ, which makes up about 2–3% of the wheat kernel, easily flakes off during milling because of its high oil content. In some milling operations, it is recovered for food use. As with wheat bran, the wheat germ can undergo further processing and refining by defatting, stabilizing, and grinding. The TDF content of wheat germ can range from 10 to 20% (12). Combining the streams during the milling process produces whole-wheat flour. Such flours contain about 12% TDF (4).

Barley. High-fiber barley ingredients have several different forms, including barley bran flour, barley flour, and barley bran. Barley bran flour is derived from barley that has been malted during the brewing process. During barley malting, the water-soluble components (sugars, starches, and β-glucan) are extracted from the grain and used in brewing. The remaining insoluble portion is then dried. This dried barley product, referred to as brewer's spent grain, is ground into what

Conditioning (also called tempering)—The addition of moisture to the kernel.

is commonly called barley bran flour. Typical levels of TDF of barley bran flour are about 50–55% and can range from 35 to 70% (13). Typically, barley bran flour is very high in insoluble fiber, with only 1–3% of the TDF present as soluble fiber (14). Barley bran flour has a malted flavor.

A hull typically covers the barley grain, but there is also a hull-less variety. Pearling is the process of removing the hull (if present), bran, and germ from the endosperm portion of the barley grain. An extensive discussion of the pearling and milling of barley is detailed elsewhere (15). The mixed bran and hull components are separated from the pearled products, which are called pot barley and pearled barley. Barley bran produced from traditional milling can have TDF levels ranging from 18 to 50% and soluble fiber of about 3–6% (15). Barley bran is not widely used in the food industry because of cost issues and a lack of development research (15). Pearled barley may be further milled into barley flour by traditional wheat milling procedures. Barley flours are relatively high in TDF and in soluble fiber. The β-glucan content of barley flours is about 3–8% (9). Typical TDF levels range up to about 10% (2). Recently, barley grain cultivars with higher fiber levels (about 38% TDF and about 15% β-glucan) have also been developed (16).

Rye. While it is not as popular as other grains in the United States, rye is a staple grain in many other countries. For instance, rye makes up about 28% of the dietary fiber intake (23 g/day) of those living in Finland (17). The milling of rye is comparable to that of other cereal grains such as wheat. High-fiber rye-based ingredients include rye bran and whole-meal rye flour. The TDF of rye bran ranges from about 15 to 30% (4). The TDF for whole rye flour is about 15% (2). Whole rye flour is reported to have more TDF than whole wheat flour, typically due to the higher *extraction rates* during milling (17).

Rice. Rice grains are processed by either of two main procedures to yield white rice or *parboiled* white rice. During both processes, the hull is removed and the remaining grain, called brown rice, is further polished by abrasion to remove the bran and germ from the endosperm. Rice bran is the high-fiber ingredient resulting from the polishing step that makes white rice or parboiled rice (Fig. 1-8). Rice bran was previously used only as pig feed in many countries because the very active lipase enzyme rapidly reacts with the oil content of the bran and germ during processing (18), causing the oil to become rancid and producing unacceptable odors and flavors. If the rice bran comes from the process for making white rice, the lipase must be inactivated immediately after polishing; this stabilizes the bran. The lipase enzyme is inactivated during the parboiling step, so there is no need for deactivation after polishing in the process for producing parboiled rice. Several technologies have been developed to produce stabilized rice bran. One involves the exposure of the bran to high temperature for a short time by using either a dry or a wet extrusion process (19). Another involves the use of the protease enzyme, which destroys the lipase enzyme (20).

Extraction rate—In the context of milling, the percentage of the intact grain recovered as flour.

Parboiled rice—Rice that has been steeped, steamed, and dried.

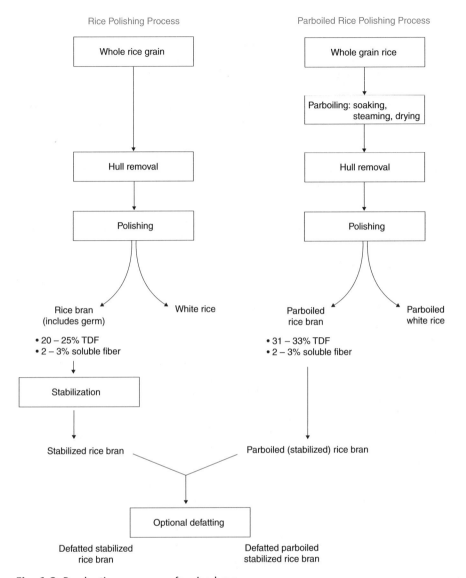

Fig. 1-8. Production processes for rice bran.

The TDF content of the rice bran ranges from 20 to 25% for straight polished rice and is 30–33% for parboiled white rice (18). Both rice bran types typically have 2–3% soluble fiber contents (18). Many rice bran producers are also able to further process the rice bran to customize the soluble/insoluble fiber content as well as the granulations of rice bran fibers.

Corn. The corn kernel is composed of the germ, the bran (often referred to as the pericarp), the endosperm, and the tip cap, which is the point of attachment of the kernel to the corncob. The germ makes up about 10–12% of the kernel by weight; the bran is about 5–6%; and the endosperm is about 80–85% (21). These components are separated by either dry milling or wet milling. Wet milling employs the use of steam or water steeping to facilitate the removal of the bran and germ. Details of the milling procedures are reviewed in detail elsewhere (21). During milling, the bran and germ components are removed in a degerminator. They are then further separated, usually by air classification.

Corn bran is the most popular high-fiber ingredient derived from corn. It is produced by the dry-milling process. The typical TDF of dry-milled corn bran is about 50–65% (4,6,21). The resulting corn bran product can undergo further refining steps such as grinding to meet particle size specifications. Further processing also leads to the removal of additional starch (22). TDF levels of refined corn brans can range from 65 to 90% (22). Of the TDF, the hemicelluloses make up about 65%, cellulose about 20%, lignin less than 0.5%, and soluble fiber less than 0.5% (21). Some manufacturers also roast the corn bran to develop nutty flavors.

Corn fiber, which is no longer available in the United States, was a corn bran product produced by the wet-milling process. This process differed from the dry-milling process in that it involved prolonged steeping of the corn kernel in water to facilitate the removal of the bran and germ from the endosperm. (Dry milling may also involve a tempering step, which is a short exposure of the kernel to steam in order to adjust the kernel moisture to about 20% [20].) Corn fiber had essentially no starch and had TDF values of about 80–95%, whereas refined corn brans contain about 4–5% starch and about 85–90% TDF.

Soybean. Two main types of high-fiber ingredients are derived from soybeans: soy hull fiber (sometimes called soy bran) and soy fiber from the cotyledon (soy endosperm). After harvest, soybeans are cleaned, cracked, dehulled, tempered, and flaked. Soy hull fiber is produced from the hull of the soybean. The hulls typically are further refined by extraction to remove lipids, etc., and the particle size may be reduced by grinding. The TDF of soy hull fiber ranges from about 65 to 95% and on average is about 75% (4,23). It is composed mainly of cellulose, an insoluble fiber. Soy fiber can also be obtained from the cotyledon and consists of both insoluble and soluble fibers. The TDF of soy fiber from the cotyledon is about 75–80% (23). Soy fiber, in contrast to soy hull fiber, is mainly composed of noncellulosic polysaccharides.

Soy protein concentrates, which can be considered a third type of high-fiber ingredient, are produced from the soy cotyledon through the extraction of soluble components such as sugars, soluble carbohydrates, and minerals. They contain about 20% TDF and about 70% soy protein, so they can be used to add both protein and fiber to foods. Soy protein concentrates contain about 14–18% insoluble fiber (mainly as hemicelluloses) and 2–6% soluble fiber (2,23).

Other grains. Amaranth, flax, spelt, and other cereal grains can also be sources of high-fiber ingredients. These grains are often available as whole-meal flours with high TDF values. In addition, some specialty processors may separate the bran and/or germ from the endosperm.

PLANT EXTRACTS OR ISOLATES

Many high-fiber ingredients are derived from plant sources other than cereal grains. These ingredients can be isolated from a variety of plant components such as the seed, woody stems, and roots. The major high-fiber ingredients derived from plant sources are discussed below.

Cellulose. Cellulose as a high-fiber ingredient is derived from sources such as wood pulp, bamboo, wheat or oat hulls, and cotton linters or cottonseeds. In general, cellulose is produced from these sources by purification to remove waxes, hemicellulose, protein, and lignin. The isolated fibers may also be bleached to remove colors. They are then dried to form a powder. Typical cellulose fiber lengths range from 22 to 290 μm (9). The fibers may also be ground to reduce their length. Different fiber lengths allow for different functionalities and help to meet certain product formulation needs, such as providing bulk (shorter fibers) or thickening (longer fibers). The TDF values of cellulose powders are very high, about 80–99%. Cellulose, which is stable to heat and pH, is most commonly used to provide bulk in formulated foods and is also used as a dusting agent to prevent clumping in foods such as shredded cheeses.

Cellulose types. It is important to understand the terminology used in referring to different types of cellulose (Box 1-2). Cellulose occurs in two forms: paracrystalline cellulose and microcrystalline cellulose (or "amorphous regions" and "crystalline regions," respectively, as mentioned earlier in the chapter). When cellulose is extracted from the plant source and is not processed further, it is called α-cellulose. Not all α-cellulose is the same, since the source can affect the size and shape of the different paracrystalline (amorphous) and microcrystalline regions, which in turn affect the final functionality of the cellulose powder. "Cellulose" and "α-cellulose" are often used interchangeably to describe the chemically unmodified high-fiber ingredient form. Cellulose gel is the product that results when α-cellulose is treated with acid to remove the paracrystalline (i.e., the amorphous, noncrystalline) regions. Despite the name, cellulose gel can exist as a free-flowing white powder. "Cellulose gel" is synonymous with "microcrystalline cellulose" (MCC), which is discussed below in the section on modified cellulose. "Cellulose gum" is the

---

Box 1-2. Cellulose Terminology

Common Term	Other Terminology	Definition
Cellulose	α-Cellulose	Pure, unmodified cellulose
Cellulose gel	Microcrystalline cellulose (MCC)	α-Cellulose treated with acid to remove amorphous regions
Cellulose gum	Carboxymethylcellulose (CMC)	Chemically modified cellulose

term commonly used for sodium carboxymethylcellulose (CMC), which is also described later in the section below.

Modified celluloses. Cellulose can be further modified, either physically or chemically, to change its functionality in foods. While there are many physical and chemical ways to modify cellulose, only a few of the resulting products are used as food ingredients.

MCC, or cellulose gel, is produced by treating α-cellulose with a mineral acid such as hydrochloric acid. It is considered an insoluble fiber. During hydrolysis, the less reactive crystalline regions of cellulose remain. The final product has a nonfibrous nature. There are many varieties of MCC available for use as food ingredients. It can exist in a powdered form, a spray-dried form, or a colloidal form. The spray-dried form is created to form aggregates with special properties. Additives such as soluble hydrocolloids (e.g., CMC or xanthan gum) are often used during spray drying so that the particles do not reaggregate during drying. MCC is often used to provide bulk and viscosity-building properties in foods such as dressings and sauces, beverages, and whipped toppings, as well as baked goods.

Methylcellulose (MC), CMC, and hydroxypropyl methylcellulose (HPMC) are all chemically modified cellulose forms called cellulose ethers. The chemical modification increases the water solubility of the cellulose. All cellulose ethers follow the same basic chemical reaction process (Fig. 1-9). Details of the reaction processes used are given elsewhere (24,25). First, cellulose is treated with a caustic solution of sodium hydroxide to yield an alkali cellulose. Treatment of the alkali cellulose with the appropriate reagent (Fig. 1-9) yields MC, CMC, or HPMC. The structures of these modified celluloses are shown in Figure 1-10. These forms are then purified to remove any residues and dried to a free-flowing powder.

Manufacturers can control the amount of substitution of the reactant onto the cellulose molecule. The amount of substitution also influences the functionalities of the final ingredient (discussed in detail in Chapter 2). MC and HPMC are cold-water soluble but are insoluble in hot water, while CMC is soluble in both cold and hot water. Food

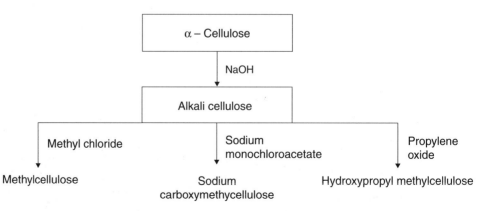

Fig. 1-9. Processing steps for the production of modified cellulose.

uses of MC include stabilization of emulsions (e.g., soups, sauces, gravies), breads, and breadings. Foods in which HPMC is used include toppings, fillings, icings, breadings, sauces, and baked goods. Foods that use CMC include frozen desserts, sauces, soups, dressings, extruded foods, and baked goods.

Gums. Plant-derived gums are soluble fibers. There are many different sources and types of gums. As described earlier in this chapter, the

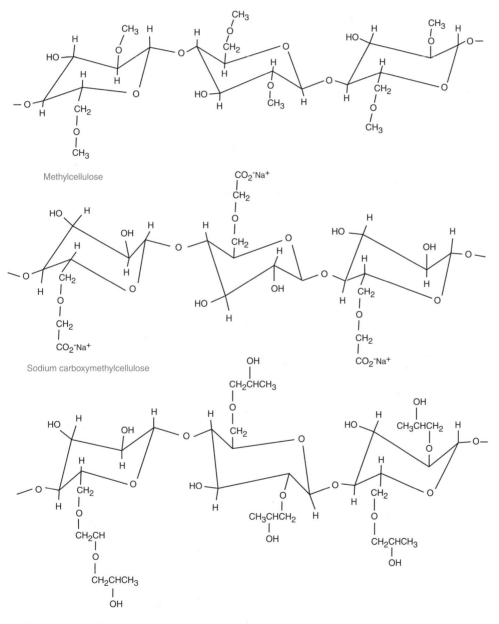

Methylcellulose

Sodium carboxymethylcellulose

Hydroxypropyl methylcellulose

Fig. 1-10. Structures of chemically modified celluloses.

components of gums are polymers that are made up of monosaccharide and uronic acid groups (Box 1-1). Because the number and functions of gums are quite extensive, the reader is referred elsewhere for a complete review. (A book on hydrocolloids, currently in preparation, is part of the Eagan Press Handbook Series.) Gums obtained from plants and commonly used in foods include seaweed extracts (carrageenan, alginates), plant extracts (gum arabic, also called gum acacia; karaya; tragacanth), and seed extracts (guar, locust bean gum). Gums obtained by microbial fermentation (e.g., xanthan, gellan) are not from plant sources but are commonly grouped with other gums.

The TDF content of gums ranges from 80 to 90%, about 98% of which is soluble (26). However, gums are not traditionally used to increase the TDF of foods because they can influence the functionality of food products at low levels (typically 0.5–2%). For example, many gums can cause a significant increase in the viscosity of the product because of their ability to bind water. Although their usage levels are often below 2% in foods, they provide many functionalities, such as viscosity, gelation, and film formation.

However, partially hydrolyzed guar gum and acacia gum can be incorporated into food formulations at levels that increase the TDF of the food without negatively affecting texture, viscosity or taste (27,28). Partially hydrolyzed guar gum has a minimum TDF of 80% and is cold-water soluble (28). Gum acacia fiber can be manufactured through a physical purification in liquid form. It is then sterilized, spray-dried, and/or granulated to produce a highly soluble white powder that is 85% TDF (29). This fiber can be used in water at levels up to 50% without greatly affecting solution viscosity (29). Both of these high-fiber ingredients are used in formulations such as beverages to increase their fiber content without significantly affecting the viscosity profile of the formulation. Since uses and use levels of gums are regulated in many countries, the formulator should check with the appropriate agency before using high levels of these gums.

Inulin and fructooligosaccharides. Inulin, a soluble fiber source, is found in more than 36,000 plants and vegetables (30). Inulin and fructooligosaccharides (FOS) are interrelated, and it is important to understand the difference in terminology. Inulin is a polymer of fructose joined by β-2-1 linkages, and it has a degree of polymerization (DP) of 2–60 units. The fructose polymers can be terminated by a glucose unit, which can provide a sweetness that is typically 0–10% that of sucrose, depending on the DP distribution (9). The DP distribution of inulin varies depending on factors such as the source and the growing conditions. Since it is a polymer of fructose, it is considered a fructan. Inulin is commercially extracted from chicory roots and is also abundant in other sources such as Jerusalem artichokes. The higher-DP forms of inulin, which are also commercially available, are less soluble and form gels at lower concentrations.

FOS are oligosaccharides of fructose containing 2–10 units of fructose that are linked by glycosidic bonds (30). Hence, they are also fructans. "Oligofructose" and "FOS" are synonymous. FOS can be produced by the partial enzymatic hydrolysis of inulin derived from chicory (30). Like inulin, FOS are linear polymers of fructose. They are typically defined as containing up to 10 fructose units. Therefore, FOS are a subcategory of inulins. Table 1-3 shows the inulin and FOS contents of various foods. Both purified inulins and FOS are commercially available and can be made with varying levels of dispersibility and solubility (discussed further in Chapter 2). The fiber content of commercially available forms of inulin and FOS is about 90%, existing as soluble fiber, with the remainder as monosaccharides and disaccharides.

Inulin is stable to heat and is easily dispersible. At pH levels less than 4, it can hydrolyze into its components of fructose and glucose. This phenomena is time and temperature dependent, with longer exposure times and higher temperatures resulting in a greater degree of hydrolysis.

Inulin has the unique ability to form gels upon being *sheared* (see Chapter 2). This property varies with the concentration of inulin (which typically needs to be >25%) and the DP of the inulin polymer chain (the longer the chain, the less inulin needed to form a gel). This unique property allows for the use of inulin to replace fat in foods such as yogurts, cheese spreads, and frozen desserts.

TABLE 1-3. Inulin and Oligofructose Contents of Various Sources[a]

Food Source	Inulin, %	Oligofructose, %
Wheat	1–6	1–4
Onion	2–10	2–6
Garlic	9–11	3–6
Jerusalem artichoke	16–20	16–20
Chicory	15–20	5–10

[a] Adapted from (7) and (36).

Konjac flour. Konjac flour is isolated from the tubers of the plant genus *Amorphophallus* (also called the Konjac plant). It has been used in traditional Japanese cooking for more than 2,000 years and is called *Konnyaku* in Japan (31). Konjac flour is a soluble dietary fiber consisting mainly of glucomannans (i.e., glucose and mannose linked in a β-1,4 linkage). These are slightly branched polymers with side chains that aid the flour's solubility properties. They have a high molecular weight (typically 200,000–2,000,000). The general isolation procedure involves grinding and milling the Konjac tuber followed by separation, washing, and drying. Konjac flour is approximately 95% TDF, more than 95% of which is soluble fiber (25). It is known for its ability to form gels in the presence of heat and alkaline conditions and also for its ability to swell and build viscosity at low levels of use. These properties are useful for the production of surimi and other meat-analog products.

Resistant starch. Resistant starches were defined earlier in the insoluble fiber section of this chapter. They are either isolated or produced for use as high-fiber ingredients in various ways. Typically, the commercial production of these ingredients involves either the isolation of RS2 type starches (e.g., isolation of granular starches from potatoes, bananas, etc.) or the production of RS3 type starches (by gelatinization

Shear—The deformation in which two adjacent planes move in a given direction while remaining parallel to each other. For instance, mixing results in shear.

and retrogradation). Some commercially prepared resistant starches, such as RS3 starches, are developed so that they withstand the processing steps of the food product into which they are incorporated (i.e., do not lose their resistance characteristics). The TDF of commercially prepared resistant starches can range from about 1 to 40% (6).

Sugar beet fiber. Sugar beet fiber is the beet pulp remaining after water extraction of the sugar from the sliced beet tuber. The pulp is dried by steam or hot air and is off-white to beige in color. The isolated fiber is about 73% TDF, about one-third of which is soluble fiber, mainly pectin (26). Its functional properties differ, though, from those of pure pectin since the pectin in sugar beet fiber is bound in the cell wall material. The ability of sugar beet fiber to bind water is useful in the extension of freshness of bread and related products. In comminuted meat applications, sugar beet fiber is used to retain the meat juice (reduce cooking losses) and as a texturizer. Sugar beet fiber is available in many dry forms from flakes to very fine particles. The fine-ground fractions can be used for fat mimicking applications.

Pea fiber. The outer shells of peas are removed and ground to produce the high-fiber ingredient pea fiber. Pea fiber can vary in color from off white to light green, depending upon the pea cultivar used. The isolated fiber can be further whitened by a chemical process. Pea fiber is available in different granule sizes, which allows the manufacturer to alter the fiber's functional properties. The TDF of pea fiber typically ranges from about 75 to 82%, depending on the cultivar. About 5% of the TDF is soluble and 77% is insoluble. The water-binding properties of pea fibers are similar to those of white (wheat) flour. Pea fibers have been used as a direct replacement for flour in high-fiber bread applications.

Arabinogalactans. Arabinogalactans are highly branched polymers composed of arabinose and galactose subunits. Arabinogalactans are extracted from the pulp of western larch trees by a water-based process (32). The commercial process for isolation involves water extraction of the arabinogalactans from the chipped wood, purification, and then drying. The subunits are linked together by β-1,3 and β-1,6 linkages. Typical molecular weights of arabinogalactans range from 50,000 to 70,000. Because of their lower molecular weight and highly branched structures, they are highly water-soluble polymers and affect solution viscosities minimally. Arabinogalactan is stable over a wide pH range. Typical TDF levels range from 80 to 90.

Psyllium seed husk. Psyllium, often called plantago, is an annual herb of the family Plantaginaceae. It is grown in India, southern Europe, and the United States. The seed of the psyllium plant has an outer covering, or hull, also commonly referred to as the husk or the Ispaghula husk (33). Psyllium seed husks have the highest known level of soluble fiber (about 70%), which is roughly eight to 10 times that of oat bran. This fiber is a polymer of arabinose, galactose, galacturonic acid, and rhamnose. It is most widely known for its ability to promote laxation.

Other minor plant sources. There are other minor sources of high-fiber ingredients derived from plant sources. The hulls of cocoa beans can be ground and used as food fiber; they are high in insoluble fibers. Tomato fiber has also been made available to the food industry. Other high-fiber plant sources, such as beans (e.g., lupine bean fiber powders) and nuts, are also available.

FRUIT-BASED INGREDIENTS

Fruits are generally known as good sources of dietary fibers. The dried fruits of dates, figs, prunes, and raisins are well-known sources of high-fiber ingredients in the food industry. They are also processed into other types of ingredient such as pastes and powders. Other fiber powders are produced from fruits such as apples. Pectin, which is isolated from fruits, is also a very common ingredient.

Dates. The use of dates as a food source goes back to the very beginnings of human civilization. A fruit of the date palm tree, dates are rich in many nutrients and are an especially good source of dietary fiber. Five to six dates provide about 3 g of dietary fiber, roughly 7.5% TDF. There are more than 30 cultivars of dates grown in California alone, five of which are used mostly in commercial applications.

Many forms of dates are available for use as ingredients in foods, including pieces, purees, pastes, and powders (34). Dehydrated date pieces (also called date sugar) are available in coarse-, medium-, and fine-grind sizes. Macerated date puree is made from dates that have been pitted and ground. Date pastes are produced by grinding macerated dates and extruding them through a screen. Diced dates and extruded pieces are also produced and are typically coated with an anticaking agent such as dextrose or oat flour to keep the pieces separated. Date powders are made by grinding the dehydrated date pieces.

Figs. Figs grow, ripen, and partially dry on the fig tree (35). They are harvested after they have fallen from the tree to ensure peak ripeness. As with dates, figs are commercially available as pastes, pieces, and powders. The pastes can either contain the seeds or come as a seedless ingredient. The two fig powders available in the United States are produced by two methods that vary slightly. In both processes, the figs are first inspected by the Dried Fruit Association of California to ensure that the fruit meets the standards set forth by the State of California Marketing Order for Dried Figs. In the production of one type of fig powder, the sugar solids are removed from the figs and the liquid (containing the sugars) is separated from the remaining solid fig material. The solid is then dehydrated, milled, and packaged. This type of powder has very low sugar content, is very free flowing, and exhibits very low *hygroscopicity*. The second type of fig powder is made by freezing or dehydrating, milling, and packaging. The two

Hygroscopicity—The ability to attract and retain moisture.

processes differ in that there is no sugar removal step in the second process. Therefore, the second type of powder is very hygroscopic, and an anticaking agent may need to be added. Fig powders can range from 12 to 64% in TDF content, depending on the process used and the customer's requirements (35).

Prunes. The processing of prunes is much like that of dates and figs. Similar forms are available, including pieces, pastes, and powders. The ripened prune plum fruit is first harvested, washed, dried in a dehydrator, packed, and then stored at 21% moisture (36). The dried prunes are stored until an order is requested, at which time they can either be further hydrated, sold whole, or processed into the high-fiber ingredient types mentioned above. Dried prunes are extruded through screens to create pastes whose viscosity can be modified by using sugar alcohols or sugar syrups (36). Oil, glucose dusting, or oat flour is used to prevent agglomeration of diced prune pieces. Prune powders are produced by grinding dehydrated prunes. The typical TDF content of dried prunes is about 7.4%, about half of which is soluble fiber. Prune powders are commercially available as blends of dried prune plums with other dried fruits, for example, dried pears or apples. The TDF content of these powders can range from 15 to 18%. Roughly half of the fiber exists as soluble fiber.

Raisins. Grapes from many cultivars are commercially available for use in foods as raisins after being dried. An excellent review of raisin production, processing, and cultivars is found elsewhere (37). The typical TDF content of raisins is about 5%. Raisin paste is also available as a food ingredient. The paste is typically produced by extruding the Thompson Seedless cultivar through a fine mesh screen (37). Raisins are fairly acidic, with a pH of about 3.5–4.0 and a titratable acidity of about 1.5–2.2% (37).

Apple fiber. Apple fiber is produced from the recovered materials (i.e., pomace) remaining after juice processing. The material is dehydrated, milled, and screened to produce a high-quality, high-fiber apple powder. The composition of the final apple fiber depends mostly on the method of juice extraction. The TDF content can range from 20 to 70% but is typically about 40%. Of this, about 30% is insoluble fiber and about 10% is soluble fiber. Apple fiber is a good source of pectin, as it can consist of about 19% pectin.

Pectin. Pectin, defined as a soluble fiber, was discussed earlier in this chapter. Commercially available pectin ingredients are produced by the extraction of pectin from citrus peels or apple pomace. They are commonly used as gelling agents and thickeners. The structure of pectin is shown in Figure 1-4. The degree of *esterification* is important to pectin functionality and directly affects gel formation, as shown in Table 1-4. Typically, low-methoxy pectins (in which <50% of the molecule is esterified) form thermoreversible gels that are softer than gels from high-methoxy pectins (in which >50% of the molecule is esterified). Pectin is commercially available in forms that differ in their de-

Esterification—The reaction of a carboxylic acid with an alcohol in the presence of an inorganic acid (e.g., sulfuric acid) to form an ester.

TABLE 1-4. Influence of Degree of Esterification on Pectin Gelation

Pectin Type	Degree of Esterification, %	Gelation Requirements
Low methoxy	<50	pH 2.9–5.5, soluble solids 10–80%
High methoxy	>50	pH 2.9–3.6, soluble solids >55% (60–80%)
Slow set	50–60	
Medium set	60–75	
Rapid set	>75	

gree of esterification. In processing pectins, the methyl groups on the pectin molecules can be deesterified by the enzyme pectin methylesterase or by solutions of acid or base. The deesterified product is termed "pectic acid."

OTHER SOURCES

Chitin and chitosan. The structural composition of chitin and chitosan are discussed in the insoluble fiber section above. Chitin is commercially extracted from the shells of crab, shrimp, and other shellfish and can be converted to the more soluble form, chitosan, by treatment with a strong base. Due to its approval status, chitin is not widely used in the food industry as an ingredient. While chitin is highly insoluble, chitosan is soluble in acid solutions and is used mainly in Japan as an ingredient in cookies and noodles.

Curdlan. Curdlan is a β-D-1,3-linked polymer of glucose. Therefore, it is a β-glucan. Curdlan, however, is an insoluble β-glucan. (Note that soluble β-glucans have mixed β-D-1,3 and -1,4 linkages.) Curdlan is greater than 90% insoluble fiber and is produced by a patented bacterial fermentation process (38) that involves isolation of curdlan by dilution with base, separation, further purification, and drying. The unique property of curdlan is that it is able to form a strong, elastic, heat-stable gel with heat. It is commonly used in Japan in the production of noodles.

Polydextrose. Polydextrose is a nonsweet bulking polysaccharide used in some food products. It is a polymer of glucose that also contains sorbitol and citric acid in an 89:10:1 mixture. A representative structure for polydextrose is shown in Figure 1-11. Polydextrose is considered either a resistant oligosaccharide or a resistant polysaccharide (resistant to alimentary enzyme degradation) and is used as a source of dietary fiber in many countries (39). Recent developments in polydextrose manufacturing have resulted in improvements in its flavor profile. Versions now have a more neutral flavor, with less acidic and bitter characteristics. Previous problems with sucrose inversion and lipid rancidity can therefore be avoided. Polydextrose is available in either a solid or liquid form. It is very water soluble and stable in solution. Suppliers can provide the form and appropriate variety for a given formulation. It is commonly used as a bulking agent

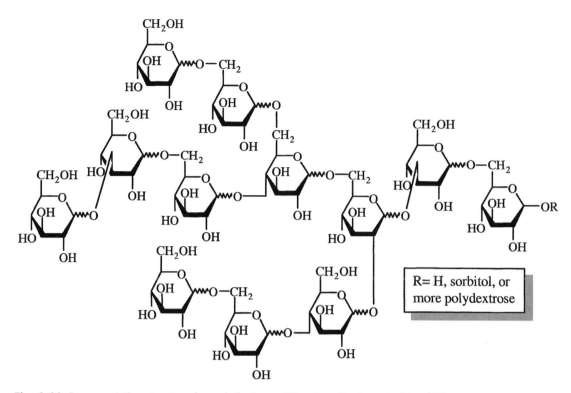

R= H, sorbitol, or more polydextrose

Fig. 1-11. Representative structure for polydextrose. (Courtesy Danisco, Ardsley, NY)

to replace sugar and/or fat in foods such as baked goods, frozen desserts, beverages, and confections.

As described in this chapter, many different types of high-fiber ingredients are available in the food industry. In addition, several factors contribute to the variability within this category. The location, growing conditions, and harvesting conditions of the source can influence the characteristics of the ingredient and its functionality. The availability, as well as other factors such as cost, may also vary depending on season or location. In addition, new research and development have led to new sources and types of high-fiber ingredients. Therefore, it is difficult to summarize every aspect of each of these ingredients. This book gives an overview of high-fiber ingredients and attempts to give the perspective needed to understand this category of ingredient. Table 1-5 summarizes the ingredients discussed in this book, along with their major sources and typical fiber ranges.

TABLE 1-5. Summary of High-Fiber Ingredients

Source Category	Source Type	Ingredient	Typical TDF[a] Range (%)
Cereal grains	Oats	Whole oats/flour	~14
		Oat fiber	80–99
		Oat bran	16–32
		Other oat ingredients (high β-glucan)	~10–15
	Wheat	Whole wheat/flour	~12
		Wheat bran	34–45
		Wheat germ	10–20
	Barley	Barley flour	~10
		Barley bran	18–50
		Barley bran flour/brewer's spent grain	35–70
	Rye	Whole rye flour	15–17
		Rye bran	~25
	Rice	Rice bran	20–35
	Corn	Corn bran	50–65
	Soy	Soy hull fiber	65–95
		Soy cotyledon fiber	~75
		Soy protein concentrate	~20
	Other grains	Amaranth, flax seed, spelt, kamut, etc.	10–15
Plant-derived	Bamboo, wood, cottonseed, etc.	Cellulose	80–99
	Modified cellulose	Microcrystalline cellulose	80–99
		Methylcellulose	80–99
		Sodium carboxymethylcellulose	80–99
		Hydroxypropyl methylcellulose	80–99
	Gums		
	Seaweed extracts	Carrageenan, alginates	80–90
	Plant extracts	Gum acacia (gum arabic), gum karaya, tragacanth gum	80–90
	Seed extracts	Guar gum, locust bean gum	80–90
	Microbially fermented	Xanthan, gellan, pullan	80–90
	Chicory roots, Jerusalem artichoke, etc.	Inulin and fructooligosaccharides	~90
	Konjac tuber	Konjac flour	~95
	Peas, outer shell	Pea fiber	75–85
	Potatoes, corn, etc.	Resistant starch	1–40
	Sugar beets	Sugar beet fiber	~75
	Western larch tree	Arabinogalactan	~80–95
	Psyllium seed coat	Psyllium	~80
Fruits	Prunes, dates figs, raisins	Whole or fruit pieces	5–8
		Powder	10–65
	Apple, pear	Powder	20–70
	Apple, citrus	Pectin	50–80
Other	Shellfish	Chitin/chitosan (modified chitin)	~80
	Bacterial fermentation	Curdlan (insoluble β-glucan)	~95
	Synthetically produced	Polydextrose	~95

[a] Total dietary fiber.

References

1. DeVries, J. W., Prosky, L., Li, B., and Cho, S. 1999. A historical perspective on defining dietary fiber. Cereal Foods World 44:367-369.
2. Cho, S., DeVries, J. W., and Prosky, L. 1997. *Dietary Fiber Analysis and Applications*. AOAC International, Gaithersburg, MD.
3. McDougall, G. J., Morrison, I. M., Stewart, D., and Hillman, J. R. 1996. Plant cells walls as dietary fiber: Range, structure, processing, and function. J. Sci. Food Agric. 70:133-150.
4. Dreher, M. L. 1987. *Handbook of Dietary Fiber: An Applied Approach*. Marcel Dekker, New York.
5. Robutti, J. L., Hoseney, R. C., and Wasson, C. E. 1974. Modified *opaque-2* corn endosperms. II. Structure viewed with a scanning electron microscope. Cereal Chem. 51:173-180.
6. Yue, P., and Waring S. 1998. Resistant starch in food applications. Cereal Foods World 43:690-695.
7. Webster, F. H., Ed. 1986. *Oats: Chemistry and Technology*. American Association of Cereal Chemists, St. Paul, MN.
8. Wood, P. J., Ed. 1993. *Oat Bran*. American Association of Cereal Chemists, St. Paul, MN.
9. Cho, S., Prosky, L., and Dreher, M. L. 1999. *Complex Carbohydrates in Foods*. Marcel Dekker, New York.
10. Hegenbart, S. 1992. Grain-based ingredients. Food Product Design 2(4):20-40.
11. Bass, E. J. 1988. Wheat flour milling. Pages 1-68 in *Wheat: Chemistry and Technology*, 3rd ed., Vol. II. Y. Pomeranz, Ed. American Association of Cereal Chemists, St. Paul, MN.
12. Vetter, J. L. 1988. Commercially available fiber ingredients and bulking agents. AIB Tech. Bull. 10(5):1-5.
13. Chaudhary, V. K., and Weber, F. E. 1990. Dietary fiber ingredients obtained by processing brewer's dried grain. J. Food Sci. 55:551, 553.
14. Lupton, J., Clayton Robinson, M., and Morin, J. 1994. Cholesterol-lowering effect of barley bran flour and oil. JAMA 94(1):65-70.
15. MacGregor, A., and Bhatty, R., Eds. 1993. *Barley: Chemistry and Technology*. American Association of Cereal Chemists, St. Paul, MN.
16. LaBell, F. 1998. Higher-fiber barley. Prepared Foods 167:91.
17. Bach Knudsen, K. E., Johansen, H. N., and Glitso, V. 1997. Rye dietary fiber and fermentation in the colon. Cereal Foods World 42:690-694.
18. Saunders, R. M. 1990. The properties of rice bran as a foodstuff. Cereal Foods World 35:632-635.
19. Hargrove, K. L., Jr. 1994. Processing and utilization of rice bran in the United States. Pages 381-404 in: *Rice Science and Technology*. W. E. Marshall and J. I. Wadsworth, Eds. Marcel Dekker, New York.
20. Deis, R. C. 1997. Functional ingredients from rice. Food Product Design 6(10):45-56.
21. Watson, S. A., and Ramstad, P. E., Eds. 1987. *Corn: Chemistry and Technology*. American Association of Cereal Chemists, St. Paul, MN.
22. Burge, R. M., and Duensing, W. J. 1989. Processing and dietary fiber ingredient applications of corn bran. Cereal Foods World 34:535-538.
23. Lo, G. 1989. Nutritional and physical properties of dietary fiber from soybeans. Cereal Foods World 34:530-534.
24. Zecher, D., and Van Coillie, R. 1992. Cellulose derivatives. Pages 40-65 in: *Thickening and Gelling Agents for Food*. A. Imeson, Ed. Chapman and Hall, New York.

25. Coffey, D. G., Bell, D. A., and Henderson, A. 1995. Cellulose and cellulose derivatives. Pages 123-153 in *Food Polysaccharides and Their Applications*. A. Stephen, Ed. Marcel Dekker, New York.
26. Deis, R. 1999. Dietary fiber: A healthy discussion. Food Product Design 8(10):97-115.
27. Greenberg, N. A., and Sellman, D. 1998. Partially hydrolyzed gum as a source of fiber. Cereal Foods World 43:703-707.
28. Novartis Nutrition. The choice is clear—Benefiber. (Tech. brochure) Novartis Nutrition—Industrial Products Division, Minneapolis, MN.
29. Colloides Naturels, Inc. 1996. FIBREGUM—A bioactive natural soluble fiber from acacia. Tech. Bull. S30/C. Colloides Naturels, Inc., Bridgewater, NJ.
30. Tungland, B. 1997. Inulin—A Healthy Functional Food Ingredient. (Report, version 25-1.5.00.) Imperial Sensus, LLC, Sugar Land, TX.
31. Kyoei Konnyaku, Inc. 2000. Konjac flour. Web site: www.kannyaku.com
32. Larex, Inc. 2000. Larex product brochure. Larex Inc., White Bear Lake, MN.
33. Cho, S. 1998. Estimation of psyllium fiber of ready-to-eat cereals. Cereal Foods World 43:368-369.
34. Sanders, S. W. 1989. Dates in bakery foods. AIB Tech. Bull. 11(6):1-6.
35. Bamford, R. 1990. Use of figs and fig products in bakery foods. AIB Tech. Bull. 12(10):1-6.
36. Sanders, S. W. 1990. Prunes in bakery products. AIB Tech. Bull. 12(3):1-6.
37. Fagrell, E. 1992. Raisin usage in baked goods. AIB Tech. Bull. 14(4):1-8.
38. Kimura, H., Sato, S., Nakagawa, T., Nakatani, H., Matsukura, A., Suzuki, T., Asai, M., Kanamaru, T., Shibata, M., and Yamatodani, S. 1973. New thermogelable polysaccharide containing foodstuffs. U.S. patent 3,754,925.
39. Craig, S. A. S, Holden, J. F., Troup, J. P., Auerbach, M. H., and Frier, H. I. 1998. Polydextrose as soluble fiber: Physiological and analytical aspects. Cereal Foods World 43:370-375.

High-Fiber Properties and Analyses

Factors Influencing Properties

The properties of high-fiber ingredients vary widely and are influenced by many factors. First, the category itself is quite broad and encompasses ingredients from many different types of sources. In addition to the type of fiber, the type and degree of processing to produce the ingredient can create even more diversity in fiber properties. The properties of the fiber, of course, affect its functions. Fibers can function in foods by adding bulk, increasing viscosity, forming gels, and replacing or mimicking fats, as well as performing other functions. Therefore, to understand how a high-fiber ingredient will function and affect the formulation, it is important to closely examine the factors that influence its properties.

TYPE OF FIBER SOURCE

The source of the high-fiber ingredient strongly influences the properties since the structural makeup of the fiber varies with the source. As discussed in Chapter 1, different types of fibers have different structural makeups, that is, different polymeric backbones and/or side-chain units. This determines the fiber's two-dimensional structure, which influences the three-dimensional structure, i.e., how the polymer interacts with itself and other polymers. For example, because of their two-dimensional linearity, cellulose molecules interact with themselves via hydrogen bonding to form crystalline regions. This gives cellulose its strength and ability to provide plants with structural integrity. Similarly, pectin molecules can gel under various circumstances (pH, presence of calcium, soluble solids content, etc.), depending on the presence and degree of carboxyl groups present in the methyl ester of the pectin molecules. It is therefore important to understand the chemical composition and structural nature of the fiber used in the formulation. Chapter 1 details the major types and structures of the principal high-fiber ingredients used in foods.

Because fibers are polymers synthesized in nature, the fiber content can also vary within a given source. For example, different oat cultivars have a wide range of fiber, protein, fat, moisture, and ash contents (1). These variations affect the final ingredient composition, since commercial extraction processes (e.g., milling) are not complete isolation processes and cannot completely isolate the fiber itself. Therefore, because the composition varies, the functional properties, such as moisture absorption, also vary.

TYPE AND DEGREE OF PROCESSING

The type of processing used to produce high-fiber ingredients largely influences the final ingredient's functionality. Milling, bleaching, grinding, enzyme treatments, stabilization procedures, extrusion, dehydration/drying, and roasting are some of the processes that are used in the production of high-fiber ingredients. The degree to which these processes are carried out also may affect the functionality. Since each of these factors plays a role in the final product's functionality, it is important to work with the ingredient manufacturer to understand how the ingredient is made and what the manufacturer can do during the process to make the ingredient most functional for the given application. How these processes affect the properties of the various high-fiber ingredients is further discussed in the next section. A general description of the processes is given below.

Milling. Milling is the physical process of separating the bran and germ layers of cereal grains from the endosperm (see Chapter 1). The degree to which these components are separated strongly influences the final ingredient's properties. The starch and other water-absorbing components are located in the endosperm of the grain. If, during the milling process, the endosperm is not completely separated from the bran and germ, the ingredient can absorb more water because of the presence of starch. If heat is present, the starch (in the presence of water) can also gelatinize, causing an increase in viscosity.

Bleaching. High-fiber ingredients can be bleached to eliminate or reduce naturally present dark or off-colors. Bleaching is done to meet consumer requirements for a white or light-colored final food product. Chemically, bleaching is an oxidation process. Combination of the ingredient with oxygen changes the molecular structure of the compound so that it no longer produces a color.

The various chemicals that can be used to oxidize compounds vary in their oxidizing strength. Dilute hydrogen peroxide is most often used to oxidize compounds in the production of high-fiber ingredients. Organic compounds also vary in their ability to participate in the oxidation reaction process and thus to become oxidized, or bleached. Tannins and other pigments are readily oxidized. Lignins are also among the more easily oxidized compounds; the oxidation process frees the carbohydrates that are bound to lignin (2). Since many organic compounds can undergo oxidation, ingredient processors carefully monitor and control the process to ensure that the pigment compounds are bleached without altering the remainder of the organic compounds.

Grinding. Grinding is a process that reduces the particle size of the fiber powders. This involves a decrease in the length of the fibers. It is most often done to reduce the negative effects on mouthfeel, such as grittiness. However, grinding can also change the water absorption properties of the fiber and influence the dispersibility and solubility properties of the powder in water. How these properties are affected depends on the type of fiber, the other processing steps, and the extent of grinding. Generalizations regarding particle size and solubility, dispersibility, or water-binding properties cannot be made across the range of high-fiber ingredients because of the variability in the physical (i.e., pore volume of the fiber, fiber length) and chemical composition of the fibers.

Grinding can cause two types of changes in the fiber powders. First, it reduces the overall particle size, which increases the total surface area of the powder. More area is then available to make contact with water. As previously described, fibers are classified as either soluble or insoluble, and the interaction of the given fiber with water also depends on these solubility characteristics. Therefore, changing the particle size of the fiber changes its interaction with water. If the fiber is *hydrophobic* (i.e., insoluble), the increase in surface area of the powder may ultimately increase the exposure of the hydrophobic fiber to water and cause a decrease in its interaction with water. For longer insoluble fibers, such as oat fibers, reduction in particle size generally decreases the water absorption of the powder. Second, the grinding may cause a decrease in the fiber's internal pore volume. For fibers such as wheat and soy, the internal pore volume is already small, and grinding does not cause any significant changes in the water absorptivity. Changes in interaction with water are also discussed in more detail in the sections on water-binding and water-holding capacities later in this chapter.

Enzyme treatments. Manufacturers can use enzymes to hydrolyze the components and thus change the product's functionality. For example, guar gum and oat β-glucans can be hydrolyzed to decrease the viscosity of the ingredient in a food system (2). Starches present in cereal-based high-fiber ingredients may also be enzymatically hydrolyzed.

Stabilization procedures. Stabilization of food fiber ingredients is largely done to eliminate enzymatic activity that causes rancidity. Rice bran is especially unstable, and the lipase enzyme must be rapidly inactivated. Stabilization procedures usually include the use of heat to inactivate the enzyme. Rice bran is often extruded, which exposes it to heat, to eliminate the enzymatic activity.

Extrusion. Extrusion can also create additional changes in the high-fiber ingredients as a result of the shear involved. The branched chains of a food polymer are susceptible to shear forces and can be cleaved from the main polymer chain, causing a change in the functionality of the ingredient, such as a decrease in its viscosity. The soluble fiber portion may also increase, depending upon the product and the extrusion conditions (2).

Hydrophobic—"Water-hating" or nonpolar.

Dehydration or drying. Many different means are used to remove water from high-fiber ingredients to produce a stable powder. The drying or dehydration processes also depend on the raw material source. For example, prune plums are dehydrated by warm-air drying, while microcrystalline cellulose can be spray dried with other components (see Chapter 1). The method of the removal of water should be understood so that the impact on the final ingredient is known. Manufacturers of high-fiber ingredients can also vary these methods (e.g., agglomeration during spray drying) to produce the desired functions (e.g., dispersibility) in the final product.

Roasting or toasting. Roasting and toasting are processes involving high temperatures to initiate the *Maillard browning* and caramelization reactions. This causes brown pigments and nutty, toasted flavors to form, which enhance the colors and flavors of the final product. These processes can also decrease the bitterness associated with some bran products. The manufacturer can vary the amount of roasting to produce the desired ingredient. Roasting and toasting processes, however, have some other effects. They can cause more difficult dispersion and hydration of soluble fibers, and some of the final reaction products may be insoluble.

Properties of High-Fiber Ingredients

High-fiber ingredients exhibit many functional properties that influence the physiological functions of foods. In addition, these functional properties directly influence the food product's properties during processing and the final product's identity. Therefore, understanding the properties of high-fiber ingredients is essential in using these ingredients to develop food products.

SOLUBILITY

The difference between the solubility of a high-fiber ingredient and the term "soluble fiber" needs to be clarified. Soluble fiber was defined in Chapter 1 as those fibers that are soluble in aqueous solutions designed to simulate human digestive systems. The analytical methodology for the determination of soluble fiber in foods attempts to identify components using that definition. The "solubility" of high-fiber ingredients refers to the state of the ingredient in water. However, the term "soluble fiber" often is used loosely to refer to the solubility of the fiber ingredient system in water. Therefore, the meaning of the term should be understood in the context of the given situation.

If a fiber is declared soluble in water, this does not mean that it is in a completely dissolved state as in the case of glucose in water. Solubility in this case is a dispersion state of the polymer in water; the fiber molecules and other components of the fiber source that are present after processing or extraction are never completely dissolved,

Maillard browning—A series of reactions in foods, dependent on time and temperature, leading to the formation of certain end products, including brown pigments.

but rather exist in a *colloidal dispersion*. In addition, high-fiber ingredients may contain soluble fiber components but still be largely insoluble in water. For example, barley and oat flours contain the water-soluble fiber β-glucan but are not soluble ingredients themselves since they contain starch as well as other water-insoluble materials. Pectins and plant gums such as gum arabic, on the other hand, are water-soluble ingredients that are largely composed of soluble fibers.

Several structural features of carbohydrate polymers affect their solubility (3). These features are important in understanding the solubility of the components of high-fiber ingredients. They are discussed below.

Branching. Branching of the polymer backbone chain disrupts the intermolecular forces and enhances solubility. Examples of highly branched high-fiber ingredients include gum acacia and arabinogalactan.

Ionizing groups. Ionizing groups (e.g., carboxylate groups) are readily solvated by water. An example of the influence of ionizing groups is the case of pectin. As the esterification of the pectin molecule increases, the amount of ionizing groups decreases, and the solubility decreases (Fig. 2-1.)

Interunit positional bonding. Certain types of backbone bonding cause nonlinearity in the polymer, thereby decreasing the opportunity for interchain bonding and increasing the ability for solvation by water molecules. The two β-glucans, curdlan and the β-glucan found in oats, barley, etc., are good examples of how variation in types of linkages (e.g., 1,3-, 1,4-, 1,6-) can affect solubility. Curdlan is a polymer of glucose that is linked completely by β-1,3 bonds. This causes the polymer to be linear, and the curdlan polymers are able to

Colloidal dispersion—The suspension of large molecules, such as polymers, in a solution.

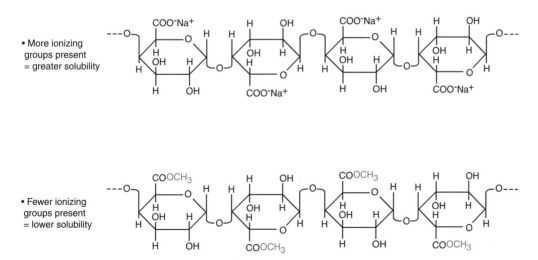

Fig. 2-1. Influence of the presence of ionizing groups on solubility of pectin. Top, before esterification; bottom, after esterification.

bond with each other. The β-glucans found in oats, barley, etc., are glucose polymers with mixed β-1,3 and β-1,4 types of linkage. This causes the β-glucan polymer to have a nonlinear nature, so the polymers are unable to extensively bond with each other and are more soluble than curdlan.

Nonuniformity. The types of monosaccharide units of the backbone chain may alternate, and/or either the α- or β-type linkages may vary. As the nonuniformity of a polymer increases, its solubility increases. Examples of soluble nonuniform polymers include gum acacia, arabinogalactan, and other gums such as xanthan gum.

The water solubilities of the high-fiber ingredients are shown in Table 2-1.

TABLE 2-1. Water Solubility of High-Fiber Ingredients

High-Fiber Ingredient	Water Insoluble	Cold-Water Soluble	Hot-Water Soluble
Cereal-based flours and brans[a]	X		
Pea fiber	X		
Cellulose	X		
Microcrystalline cellulose	X		
Resistant starch	X		
Chitin/chitosan	X		
Methylcellulose		X	
Hydroxypropyl methylcellulose		X	
Carboxymethylcellulose		X	X
Pectins		X	X
Carageenan		X	X
Alginate		X	X
Acacia		X	X
Karaya			X
Tragacanth		X	X
Guar		X	X
Locust bean gum			X
Xanthan		X	X
Gellan			X
Arabinogalactan		X	X
Inulin		X	X
Konjac flour		X	X
Sugar beet fiber[b]	X		
Psyllium seed husk[b]	X		
Date, prune, raisin, fig[b]	X		
Apple, pear[b]	X		
Curdlan	X		
Polydextrose		X	X

[a] Some cereal high-fiber ingredients contain soluble fiber components (i.e., β-glucan in oats, barley, etc.)

[b] Contains soluble fibers.

VISCOSITY

The fundamental rheological property of a fluid is known as the viscosity. High-fiber ingredients are able to contribute to the viscosities of food systems. Therefore, the basic principles of viscosity are reviewed here. Viscosity is defined as the ratio of the *shear stress* to the *shear rate*. A Newtonian fluid is one for which the viscosity remains constant for any given shear rate. Water is a Newtonian fluid. If the viscosity changes as the shear rate changes, the fluid is said to be either dilatant or pseudoplastic. Dilatant fluids increase in viscosity with increasing shear rate, while pseudoplastic fluids decrease in viscosity with increasing shear rate. For instance, heather honey is a dilatant fluid; it gets more viscous with stirring. Gelatinized starch-in-water suspensions exhibit pseudoplastic behavior because the starch molecules align with the direction of the flow, and the suspension becomes thinner. A graphical depiction of Newtonian, dilatant, and pseudoplastic fluids is shown in Figure 2-2A.

Fluid systems can also exhibit other dependencies that affect their viscosity. A plastic fluid is one that withstands a certain amount of stress before it begins to flow. This stress is called the yield stress or yield value. This phenomena is depicted in Figure 2-2B. Time dependencies of fluids are described as either thixotropic or rheopectic. If the viscosity decreases with time, the fluid is thixotropic. If the viscosity increases with time, the fluid is rheopectic. These fluid types are shown in Figure 2-2C.

Many factors affect the viscosity of high-fiber ingredients (Table 2-2). In general, as the molecular weight or fiber length of the food polymer increases, the viscosity increases. The concentration of fiber present, temperature, shear conditions, pH, and ionic strength are all factors that strongly depend on and vary widely with the type of fiber used.

Although the cereal-based high-fiber ingredients (e.g., oat flour, wheat bran, etc.), as well as the fruit-based ones and other high-fiber ingredients such as chitosan, can affect the viscosity of food products, the plant-derived gums are the most widely used as thickening agents to specifically increase the viscosity of the food. Gums such as guar and locust bean gum are also called hydrocolloids because they form colloidal dispersions in water. In general, the lowest-viscosity plant gums are gum acacia, isolated arabinogalactans, and inulin. Gum acacia does not begin to affect solution viscosities until levels of about 50% (4). Arabinogalactans exhibit the viscosity of a Newtonian fluid. Inulin does not generally begin to affect solution viscosity until concentrations of about 15–25%, depending on the chain length of the inulin polymers. Inulin can form a gel at concentrations greater than 25% inulin in water at room temperature. In general, longer chains produce firm gels at concentrations of about 35%, while shorter chains produce softer gels at this concentration. On the other hand, guar gum, tragacanth gum, and Konjac flour are the highest-viscosity plant gums and

Shear stress—The amount of a force, such as stirring, applied to a material.

Shear rate—The speed at which a force, such as stirring, is applied.

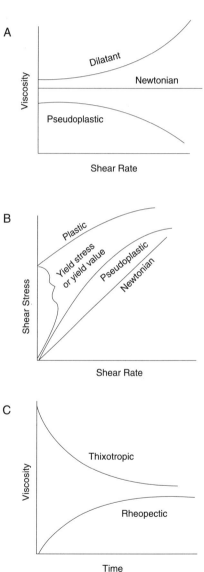

Fig. 2-2. Viscosity behavior of fluids. A, behavior of Newtonian, dilatant, and pseudoplastic fluids; B, yield stresses of fluids; C, behavior of thixotropic and rheopectic fluids.

TABLE 2-2. Factors Influencing the Viscosity of High-Fiber Ingredients

Factor	General Impact
Concentration of high-fiber ingredient	As concentration increases, viscosity increases.
Nature of polymer of high-fiber ingredient	As molecular weight increases, viscosity increases. As branching decreases (linearity increases), viscosity increases.
Presence of cereal-based starch	As cereal-based starch increases, viscosity increases.
pH	Varies with fiber type.
Ionic strength	Varies with fiber type.

TABLE 2-3. General Viscosity Characteristics of Several High-Fiber Ingredients[a]

Produce High Viscosity	Produce Low Viscosity
Konjac flour	Gum acacia
Gum tragacanth	Inulin
Guar gum	Partially hydrolyzed guar
Gum karaya	Arabinogalactan
Locust bean gum	

[a] Viscosity characteristics of cereal-based high-fiber ingredients highly depend on their processing.

exhibit high viscosities at very low concentrations. Hydrolyzed guar gum, however, produces very low viscosities in solution (5). Table 2-3 shows the viscosity characteristics of some high-fiber ingredients. An excellent review of the viscosities of the plant gums can be found elsewhere (6,7). An Eagan Press handbook on hydrocolloids is being prepared.

Viscosity measurement. Viscosity in food systems is usually measured using a rotational-type viscometer. The Brookfield and Haake viscometers are two rotational-type devices that are commonly used. The Brookfield instrument consists of a rotating spindle connected to a spring. The resistance of the force of the solution on the rotating spindle is measured via the spring. The spindle velocity and spindle type can be varied; thus, the shear rate and shear stress, respectively, can be varied. The Haake viscometer gives a very high precision, and the shear stress and shear rate can also be varied.

GELATION

Gelation can be described as the association of polymer units to form a network of junction zones. The regions within the junction zones are compartments that contain water and other solutes. The resulting gel has a three-dimensional, firm structure. Many water-soluble fibers and gums have the capability of forming gels. The plant gums are often used as gelling agents in the development of food products. Formation of the gel depends on many factors such as type of gum, concentration, temperature, presence of ions (e.g., calcium), pH, or the presence of other gums. The characteristics of the gel also depend on these factors. Table 2-4 shows the gelation conditions and characteristics of some high-fiber ingredients. Nongelling gums include guar (and partially hydrolyzed guar gum), gum arabic, karaya, lambda carrageenan, and tragacanth.

Measuring gel strength. The measurement of gel strength involves the measurement of a penetration force and the resistance of the gel to that force. Three methods are commonly used in the food industry to measure gel strength (8). The Bloom test is a widely recognized method that measures the force of deflection of a probe from the sur-

TABLE 2-4. Gelation Conditions for High-Fiber Ingredients

Gelation Condition	High-Fiber Ingredient	Gel Characteristics
Shear, water	Inulin	Gels at concentrations >25%
		Type of gel depends on the concentration and degree of polymerization (DP) of the inulin polymer. Longer chains (DP 23 units) form firm gels, while shorter chains (DP 9 units) form softer gels at about 35% inulin in water.
Heat	Curdlan	Thermoirreversible at >80°C (highset); strong, elastic
		Thermoreversible at 60°C (lowset)
	Hydoxypropyl methylcellulose	Thermoreversible
	Methylcellulose	Thermoreversible
	Pectin (high methoxy)	Needs acid conditions
Potassium ions	Kappa-carrageenan	Thermoreversible
Calcium ions	Pectin (low methoxy)	Thermoirreversible
	Iota-carrageenan	Thermoreversible
	Alginates	Thermoirreversible
	Gellan	Thermoirreversible
Alkaline conditions	Konjac flour	Strong, elastic, thermoirreversible
Other gums	Locust bean gum	Needs xanthan or kappa-carrageenan
	Xanthan gum	Needs locust bean gum or konjac flour

face of the gel to a 4-mm penetration depth without rupturing the gel. The results are expressed in Bloom or Bloom grams and can range from 30 to 300 g (8). The Bloom Gelometer should be used for softer gels. Another method, used for firmer gels such as pectin or agar gels, is similar to the Bloom method but uses a larger-diameter probe and requires that the gel actually rupture. The third test, used for very firm, rigid gels, involves cutting a cylinder out of the gel. The gel cylinder is placed between two plates that are then forced together until the gel ruptures. In both of these methods, the measurement is the force required to rupture the gel.

WATER-BINDING CAPACITY

The way in which water interacts with high-fiber ingredients can be described using many terms such as water uptake, hydration, adsorption, absorption, binding, or holding. Different suppliers or laboratories may use different terms that actually mean the same thing. On the other hand, users may have different definitions for the same term. It is very important to understand how the term is defined in each situation.

Two terms important for understanding high-fiber ingredients are "water-holding capacity" and "water-binding capacity." For the purposes of this text, the definitions given by Rey and Labuza (9) are used to distinguish the two terms. While they define these terms in the context of gels, the same principle can be applied in the area of fibers. In the context of high-fiber ingredients in this text, the terms are defined as follows:

TABLE 2-5. Water-Binding Capacity of Various High-Fiber Ingredients[a]

Ingredient	Water-Binding Capacity (g water/g material x 100)[b]
Apple pulp	230
Rice bran	100
Wheat bran	260
Oat bran	140
Corn bran	250
Soy bran	240
Sugar beet fiber	350

[a] Adapted from (14).
[b] By AACC method 56-30 (13).

Water-holding capacity (WHC): the amount of water the (gel) system retains within its structure without subjection to any given addition of pressure or stress.

Water-binding capacity (WBC): the amount of water the (gel) system retains after it has been subjected to a stress (e.g., centrifugation).

Since the manufacturing or processing of food products usually involves the use of some type of physical stress (e.g., kneading of bread dough, extrusion of cereals, homogenization of dairy products), the WBC is discussed here. Table 2-5 lists the water-binding capacity of selected high-fiber ingredients.

Numerous factors influence the WBC of high-fiber ingredients. While the raw material source is a determining factor in the WBC of the ingredient, it is not the only factor involved. This makes comparing WBC data difficult. Figure 2-3 schematically depicts the factors that influence the final WBC. Note that raw material does not solely determine the WBC of a high-fiber ingredient. It does determine the chemical and structural makeup of the high-fiber ingredient, which influences the microstructure of the ingredient. Robertson and Eastwood (10) reported that the capacity of fiber to bind water was a function of the fiber source and method of measurement and that the structure of the fiber was more influential than the chemical composition of the fiber. The fiber microstructure includes characteristics such as the fiber length, particle size, and the porosity of the ingredient. The microstructure is a function of both the raw material source and the processing conditions used in producing the high-fiber ingredient. Therefore, ingredient suppliers may have some ability to alter the WBC of their ingredients and to work with the food formulators to meet the development needs.

Another determining factor for the WBC is the food system environment. The pH, ionic strength, concentration of the high-fiber ingredient, and presence of other water-binding ingredients (i.e., sugars, starches, etc.) all have an influence on the WBC of the high-fiber ingredient. For soluble fibers, the pH and ionic strength can directly affect the fiber molecule's interaction with water. However, because of the number of determining factors (Fig. 2-3), care must be taken in comparing any WBC data of high-fiber ingredients. In addition, the method of measurement for WBC influences the final results.

Measurement of WBC. Not only are there many different terms for the WBC of a high-fiber ingredient, but there are many different methods of measurement and no

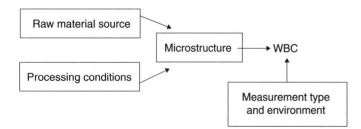

Fig. 2-3. Factors determining water-binding capacity (WBC).

internationally recognized standard method. This can make comparisons of WBC data difficult, and care should be taken when comparing data from different sources. Recently, a collaborative study involving several hydration properties of fibers resulted in the development of a standardized centrifugation-based method to approximate WBC (11). Good statistical results were achieved for samples of resistant starch, pea hull, citrus pulp, and apple pulp.

Generally, the methods for measuring WBC involve the addition of a volume of water to a sample and then measurement of the entrapped or held water after the free water has been separated from the sample. The water is separated either by filtration, centrifugation, or dialysis. Exact conditions (e.g., temperature) should be stated for the method since WBC depends on many variables. A complete review of the direct and indirect methods (including sorption isotherm techniques and freezing point depression) for measuring WBC and WHC can be found elsewhere (12). Brief descriptions of the methods commonly used are discussed below.

Centrifugation methods. Centrifugation methods are widely used by high-fiber ingredient manufacturers. The AACC method (56-30) is based on centrifugal separation of the free water from the sample (13). First, water is added to 5 g of sample. The sample is then centrifuged at $2,000 \times g$ for 10 min. The supernatant is discarded, and the remaining sediment is weighed. The difference between the wet and dry weights is calculated as the water hydration capacity (a term used in the same way as WBC). This method is often used for the WBC of insoluble fibers such as corn bran and oat fibers. Modifications to the method are often made by varying the sample amount, water amount, and/or centrifugation conditions (12,14,15).

Dialysis methods. These methods were developed to mimic the physiological conditions that the fiber encounters during digestion. They are also used for water-soluble fibers that cannot be centrifuged, such as guar gum. The sample is put into semipermeable dialysis tubing and placed into a solution that mimics the human intestinal system. Since there is no physical stress involved, the dialysis methods measure the WHC, which is calculated as the amount of weight gained by the tube after immersion (12,14,15).

OIL-BINDING CAPACITY

Dietary fibers are also known to bind oil. While the chemical composition of the fiber itself plays a role, the ability to bind oil is more a function of the porosity of the fiber structure than of the affinity of the fiber molecule for oil (as in the case of WBC). Presoaking a high-fiber ingredient with water can help to reduce the amount of oil pickup by the ingredient since the water occupies the pores in the fiber before the oil is added. This phenomenon is useful in the formulation of batters and breadings to reduce the uptake of oil during frying and decrease the total fat of the fried food product. Also, in formulating comminuted or emulsified meat, the addition of fiber can

Cations—Positively charged ions.

Cation-exchanger—A polymer with the ability to selectively bind and release charged molecules (minerals, monomers, and polymers) under different conditions of acidity or salt concentration.

enhance the emulsion by retaining the fat present in the formula. In low-fat meat applications, this function is important in that the fiber retains the low amount of fat present, which aids the texture and juiciness of the final cooked product.

MINERAL AND ORGANIC MOLECULE BINDING

Because of the presence of uronic acids as well as the free carboxyl groups of the component monosaccharides, many dietary fibers are able to bind *cations* such as calcium, cadmium, zinc, and copper. A notable example of this phenomenon is pectin. At acidic pH levels, low-methoxy pectins are able to bind calcium ions, which aids in forming a gel structure. Wheat bran is considered a weak *cation-exchanger*. The ability to bind positively charged materials, such as some minerals, to fiber components is known as the cation exchange capacity (CEC) and is described elsewhere (12,14,15). Factors that influence the CEC include type of fiber, pH, ionic strength, and nature of the cation (15). An exception to mineral binding is the ability of some soluble fibers such as inulin and oligofructose to increase the bioavailability of minerals such as calcium, magnesium, and iron (16).

Dietary fibers have also been shown to absorb certain organic molecules. The absorption is also dependent on the pH of the system. For example, lignin can bind bile acids, while wheat bran can bind carcinogens such as benzopyrazine (12). The absorption of organic molecules such as carcinogens is important to the physiological function of dietary fibers. This property is believed to reduce the risk of certain cancers.

Fiber Analyses

Several methods have been developed to assess dietary fiber and its components. The history of this development was also addressed in Chapter 1. The methods for dietary fiber analysis are found in the *Approved Methods of the American Association of Cereal Chemists*, which is published by the AACC, as well as in the *Official Methods of Analysis*, which is published by AOAC (Association of Official Analytical Chemists) International. These texts are revised and updated periodically and printed as new editions. Methods from both books are usually referenced or cited in the literature by their method number. For example, the total dietary fiber method is listed as AACC 32-05 or AOAC 985.29 (17,18). Methods for dietary fiber are classified into three categories (12): 1) nonenzymatic-gravimetric, 2) enzymatic-gravimetric, and 3) enzymatic-chemical.

For a complete review of all of the methods described here, as well as their history, the reader is referred to references 2, 12, and 19.

The nonenzymatic-gravimetric methods are those that were developed early on to determine total dietary fiber. These include the crude fiber (CF) method (AACC 32-10/AOAC 920.86), the acid detergent fiber (ADF) method (no approved AACC/AOAC methods), and the neutral detergent fiber (NDF) methods (no approved AACC/AOAC methods). The CF, ADF, and NDF methods are not widely used for food labeling in the United States since they do not determine all of the components that are now considered part of the total dietary fiber definition. The CF method measures lignin and cellulose; the ADF method measures lignin, cellulose, and acid-insoluble hemicelluloses; and the NDF method measures lignin, cellulose, and the neutral detergent-insoluble residues (12).

The enzymatic-gravimetric methods, which are the more common methods used to identify the fiber components for food labeling of high-fiber ingredients, are discussed below.

TOTAL DIETARY FIBER

While any of the approved methods for total dietary fiber may be used for nutritional labeling purposes in the United States, the most widely used and currently accepted method for dietary fiber is the enzymatic-gravimetric method. This is AACC method 32-05 or AOAC method 985.29 (17,18). Basically, the method involves defatting the sample (if it contains more than 10% fat) and then removing the digestible portions of the sample through the use of enzymes. The remaining, nondigestible portions are then precipitated with ethanol, dried, weighed, and corrected for protein and ash content. The consistency, precision, and accuracy of the method highly depend on the purity of the enzyme system used as well as the digestion step (19). A current issue with this method is that it does not include components such as resistant starch, nondigestible oligosaccharides such as inulin, fructooligosaccharides, and polysaccharides such as polydextrose, even though these components have been found to have the physiological effects of dietary fiber. Other methods have been developed to assay for these missing components. The key methods for components related to dietary fiber are listed in Table 2-6.

SOLUBLE/INSOLUBLE DIETARY FIBER

The AACC 32-05/AOAC 985.29 method was later modified in order to isolate the important fractions of soluble and insoluble fibers. The modified method (AACC 32-07/AOAC 991.43) is also an enzymatic-gravimetric assay. The insoluble dietary fiber is filtered and washed with water. The solution of the filtrate and the water washings are precipitated in 78% ethanol, which is then filtered and dried in order to determine the soluble dietary fiber. The insoluble dietary fiber and soluble dietary fiber are determined gravimetrically, correcting for the protein and ash components. The total dietary fiber can also be calculated using this method.

The enzymatic-chemical methods are similar to the enzymatic-gravimetric methods, but they further break down the fiber molecules in order to quantify components such as uronic acids, lignin, and monosaccharides. The uronic acids can be quantified using colorimetric or decarboxylation methods; the lignin is gravimetrically determined using the Klason lignin procedure; and the monosaccharides can be quantified using gas chromatography or high-performance

TABLE 2-6. Key Methods for Determining Components of Dietary Fiber

Method Numbers	Description	Comments
AACC 32-05 AOAC 985.29	Measures total dietary fiber in foods by an enzymatic-gravimetric method	Does not quantitate soluble fibers that are soluble in 78% ethanol (e.g., inulin, poly-dextrose, fructooligosaccharides, and other oligosaccharides)
AACC 32-21 AOAC 991.42	Measures insoluble dietary fiber in foods by an enzymatic-gravimetric method with a phosphate buffer	Soluble fiber can be determined by utilizing both AOAC 985.29 and AOAC 991.42
AACC 32-21 AOAC 993.19	Measures soluble dietary fiber in foods by an enzymatic-gravimetric method with a phosphate buffer	Total dietary fiber can be determined by utilizing AOAC methods 991.42 and 993.19 together
AACC 32-07 AOAC 991.43	Measures total, soluble, and insoluble dietary fiber in foods by an enzymatic-gravimetric method with a MES-Tris[a] buffer	Does not quantitate soluble fibers that are soluble in 78% ethanol (e.g., inulin, poly-dextrose, fructooligosaccharides, and other oligosaccharides)
AOAC 2000.11	Measures polydextrose in foods	
AACC 32-32 AOAC 997.08	Measures fructans in foods by ion exchange chromatography	For determination of inulin in foods
AACC 32-22 and 32-23 AOAC 992.28 and 995.16	Measures β-D-glucan component in cereals	

[a] 2(*N*-morpholino)ethanesulfonic acid plus tris(hydroxymethyl)-animomethane.

liquid chromatography. Cho et al describe the complete procedures for each of these methods (12).

Ingredient Specifications

Ingredient specification sheets are provided to the ingredient purchaser by the supplier. They are a compilation of the quality requirements of the ingredient that the food manufacturer, or buyer, specifies. The specifications can vary from supplier to supplier and depend on what the buyer requires. Specification sheets for high-fiber ingredients usually contain the following information.

Product description. This can be as simple as the product name. It also can include a brief paragraph describing the manufacturing process, composition, and form of the ingredient. Kosher status can also be listed as part of the specification.

Physical data. Physical data such as appearance, flavor/taste, color, and aroma are often listed and are straightforward in their meaning. Other physical data that may be specified for high-fiber ingredients are defined below.

Bulk density. The bulk density is the mass per unit volume of the high-fiber ingredient as it is normally packed (i.e., not compressed), with the void spaces between the particles containing air. It is expressed as lb/ft^3 or g/cm^3. For a given high-fiber powder, the higher the bulk density value, the more closely the particles are packed together and the more "dense" the powder.

pH. For a high-fiber ingredient, the pH is usually given for a mixture of the ingredient in water. The percentage of ingredient in water as well as the temperature of the measurement should be noted.

Viscosity. The measurement of viscosity was discussed earlier in this chapter. The specification should list the method and conditions used for measurement.

Particle size/granulation. There are many methods for determining the particle size or granulation of powders. Particle size distributions of the powders can also be measured and listed on the specifications. Again, the methods used to determine this should be listed.

Water-holding properties. The water-absorption, -hydration, or -binding properties of the ingredients can be specified and also highly depend on the method and conditions used.

Chemical data. The chemical data reported usually include the moisture, protein, fat, ash, carbohydrate, fiber, calories, and vitamin and mineral contents of the ingredient. The fiber content may include the total, soluble, and insoluble portions. Other components of the fiber can also be listed, such as the crude fiber, lignin, cellulose, and hemicellulose components. The enzyme activity can also be listed in this section (usually measured as peroxidase activity).

Microbiological tests. The required microbiological tests are specified in this section. Typical tests include standard plate count (or total aerobic plate count), yeasts, molds, *Bacillus cereus*, coliforms, *Staphylococcus aureus*, *Salmonella*, and *E. coli* and are usually noted with the acceptable results.

Packaging/shelf life/storage. This section describes how the ingredient supplier packages the ingredient, what the typical shelf life of the ingredient is, and the recommended means of storing the ingredient. This can vary with the supplier and type of high-fiber ingredient purchased.

References

1. Wood, P. J. 1993. *Oat Bran.* American Association of Cereal Chemists, St. Paul, MN.
2. Cho, S., Prosky, L., and Dreher, M. L. 1999. *Complex Carbohydrates in Foods.* Marcel Dekker, New York.
3. Glass, J. E. 1986. Water solubility in carbohydrate polymers. Pages 3-27 in: *Water Soluble Polymers—Beauty with Performance.* J. E. Glass, Ed. Advances in Chemistry Series 213. American Chemical Society, Washington, DC.
4. Colloides Naturels, Inc. July, 1996. FIBREGUM—A bioactive natural soluble fiber from acacia. Tech. Bull. S30/C. Colloides Naturels, Inc., Bridgewater, NJ.
5. Silva, R. F. 1996. Use of inulin as a natural texture modifier. Cereal Foods World 41:792-794.
6. Ward, F. M., and Andon, S. A. 1993. Water-soluble gums used in snack foods and cereal products. Cereal Foods World 38:748-752.

7. Stephen, A. M. 1995. *Food Polysaccharides and Their Applications*. Marcel Dekker, New York.

8. Pryzbyla Wilkes, A. 1992. Evaluating gel strength. Food Product Design 1(12):59-64.

9. Rey, D. K., and Labuza, T. P. 1981. Characterization of the effect of solutes on the water-binding and gel strength properties of carageenan. J. Food Sci. 46:786-789.

10. Robertson, J. A., and Eastwood, M. A. 1981. An examination of factors which may affect the water holding capacity of dietary fibre. Br. J. Nutr. 45(1):83-88.

11. Robertson, J. A., de Monredon, F. D., Dysseler, P., Guillon, F., Amado', R., and Thibault, J. F. 2000. Hydration properties of dietary fibre and resistant starch: A European collaborative study. Lebensm. Wiss. Technol. 33:72-79.

12. Cho, S., DeVries, J. W., and Prosky, L. 1997. *Dietary Fiber Analysis and Applications*. AOAC International, Gaithersburg, MD.

13. AACC. 2000. *Approved Methods of the American Association of Cereal Chemists*, 10th ed. Method 56-30, Water hydration capacity of protein materials. The Association, St. Paul, MN.

14. Dreher, M. L. 1987. *Handbook of Dietary Fiber: An Applied Approach*. Marcel Dekker, New York.

15. Thibault, J. F., Lahaye, M., and Guillon, F. 1992. Physico-chemical properties of food plant cell walls. Pages 21-56 in: *Dietary Fibre—A Component of Food: Nutritional Function in Health and Disease*. T. F. Schweizer and C. A. Edwards, Eds. Springer-Verlag, Berlin.

16. Tungland, B. 1997. Inulin—A Healthy Functional Food Ingredient. Version 25-1.5.00. Imperial Sensus, LLC. Sugar Land, TX.

17. AACC. 2000. *Approved Methods of the American Association of Cereal Chemists*, 10th ed. Method 32-05, Total dietary fiber. The Association, St. Paul, MN.

18. AOAC International. 1995. *Official Methods of Analysis*, 16th ed. AOAC Official Method 985.29. Total dietary fiber in foods—Enzymatic-gravimetric method. The Association, Gaithersburg, MD.

19. DeVries, J. W., Prosky, L., Li, B., and Cho, S. 1999. A historical perspective on defining dietary fiber. Cereal Foods World 44:367-369.

Baked Goods and Extruded Applications

Of all the categories of food products, the most common fiber-enriched products are the baked and extruded grain products. High-fiber breads and cereals are widely available and are consumed as a means of meeting the recommended amounts of dietary fiber in the daily diet. While these products are now widely available, many obstacles were encountered during their development. Consumers found the texture and flavor of many of the first high-fiber breads unpleasant. In addition, when consumers became aware that cellulose, one of the first high-fiber ingredients used in breadmaking, was derived from wood sources, the term "sawdust" became associated with these breads. However, new developments in high-fiber ingredients have allowed processors to formulate good-tasting, consumer-accepted high-fiber bread products. Although problems with product shapes and bowl-life still exist with many high-fiber extruded cereals, improvements have been made and the products have become accepted by consumers. High-fiber ingredients have also become widely used in this product category as a means of decreasing the fat and calorie content of these foods.

Breads and Related Products

Breads encompass a wide variety of products, including white bread, rye bread, whole-grain varieties such as whole wheat or multigrain bread, and other variety and specialty breads. Bagels, English muffins, rolls, and buns are also considered to be in the bread category since they rely on similar processing steps and ingredients.

To understand how high-fiber ingredients affect the processing and quality of the final bread or related product, it is important to understand the general aspects of the breadmaking process. Wheat flour, typically the main ingredient in bread, consists primarily of starch and some protein. During the mixing and kneading of bread doughs, the protein components gliadin and glutenin combine in the presence of water to form a gluten matrix. The gluten is responsible for the elastic properties of the dough, and it retains the gas produced during fermentation, which allows the bread to rise.

All yeast-raised bread processes include mixing, fermentation, and baking steps. Mixing creates a homogeneous mass of all the ingredients. During mixing, the water in the formula hydrates the

Dough strengthener— Material (e.g., sodium stearyl lactylate or ethoxylated mono-glycerides) added to bread dough to increase the ability of the gluten to retain gas during proofing and baking.

Sponge—In breadmaking, a mixture of water, yeast, yeast food, and part of the flour, which is mixed separately in order to combine these ingredients without forming the gluten matrix.

Molding—In baking, the step in which the dough is formed into the desired shape.

Proofing—A step in preparing yeast-leavened products in which the dough is warmed and allowed to rise. It takes place after an initial fermentation and before baking.

ingredients; the starches swell; and the gluten matrix forms, causing the dough to develop. If the dough is overmixed, it becomes too extensible and sticky. During fermentation, the yeasts metabolize the sugars, forming gas that is retained within the dough. During baking, the dough expands further; the starch gelatinizes; and a solid structure is formed. Additives are sometimes used in breadmaking to aid in the proper development of the dough and final product. For example, the addition of oxidizing agents (e.g., ascorbic acid, potassium bromate, or azodicarbonamide) can help the proteins of the flour to form gluten. Added emulsifiers such as sodium stearyl lactylate (SSL) or ethoxylated monoglycerides can improve loaf quality and volume by acting as *dough strengtheners* and aiding in the development of gluten (1).

There are several breadmaking processes, which are described elsewhere (2). The process commonly used in commercial production of bread is called the sponge-and-dough method. This involves the formation of a *sponge*, which is then fermented. After the fermentation, the sponge is described as either plastic or liquid, depending on its consistency. The remaining ingredients are then added to the sponge and mixed until the dough is fully developed. Dough development is highly dependent on both the mixing time and the water absorption properties of the ingredients that make up the dough. The dough is then *molded*, *proofed*, and baked.

Several instruments, e.g., the mixograph, farinograph, extensigraph, and amylograph, can be used to predict the mixing behaviors of doughs. The most commonly used instruments, the farinograph and the mixograph, measure the work and time required to mix dough to the proper consistency. The amount of water used to reach this condition is also noted by these devices, and they are therefore used to measure the water absorption of flour. The extensigraph measures dough elasticity by recording the amount of force used to stretch the dough. The amylograph measures batter viscosity and is used to measure how the ingredients in a dough system absorb water when heated.

ADDITION OF FIBER TO BREAD

Breads are sources of carbohydrates and can also be sources of dietary fiber. The dietary fiber content of various breads is shown in Table 3-1. High-fiber ingredients are added to breads for several reasons. First, they are used to increase the total dietary fiber (TDF) content of the bread. Second, they can be used to decrease the calories in the bread. High-fiber ingredients such as inulin, psyllium, apple fiber, or sugar beet fiber can also improve the perception of freshness. Common high-fiber ingredients used for high-fiber and low-calorie breads and related products include whole grains and whole-grain flours, cereal fibers and brans (e.g., oat [hull] fiber, wheat bran, and rice bran), germ (e.g., wheat germ), and celluloses. These sources contain higher amounts of insoluble fibers than soluble fibers.

For labeling purposes in the United States, insoluble fibers contribute zero calories per gram, while soluble fibers contribute four calories per gram. Therefore, fiber sources that are high in both TDF and insoluble fiber are usually preferred when formulating reduced-calorie breads. Such breads are defined as having one-third fewer calories than their full-calorie counterparts. (A white bread formula [Table 3-2] is usually used as the standard reference.) It has been reported that the TDF of the fiber source should be about 70% and that the fiber should replace about 30% of the flour, using a typical white bread formula as the basis of the reduced-calorie formula. Any fat source should be removed; there should be a 10–15% addition of vital wheat gluten; and the moisture content should be increased 4–6% (3). The moisture content of reduced-calorie breads is often as high as 43–45% because of the addition of the fiber.

The formulation of a high-fiber or reduced-calorie bread involves the substitution of the high-fiber ingredient for a portion of the flour. The amount substituted depends on the desired labeling of the final product as well as on the high-fiber ingredient(s) used. It can range from a fraction of a percent to as high as 20% for a reduced-calorie product.

Each high-fiber ingredient affects the breadmaking process and the final products in different ways. Substitution levels of fiber ingredients such as soy bran, pea fiber, cocoa hulls, coffee hulls, and sugar beet fiber at levels greater than 20% have resulted in poor-quality breads (4,5). In general, typical additions for high-fiber (full-calorie) bread range from about 1 to 10% (3,5,6). For a typical serving of 50 g (approximately one slice of bread), a TDF of the final product of 5% would result in a labeling declaration of 2.5 g of fiber per serving. Usage levels of the insoluble fiber types (such as cellulose or wheat bran) of 7–7.5% provide the best-quality breads, with higher fiber contents than white bread and minimal processing changes (3,6).

TABLE 3-1. Dietary Fiber Content (%) of Various Breads[a]

Bread	Dietary Fiber		
	Total	Soluble	Insoluble
Bran	5.4	4.6	0.8
Cracked wheat	5.3	4.5	0.8
French	2.7	1.9	0.8
Multigrain	5.6	4.6	1.0
Oatmeal	4.3	3.3	1.0
Reduced-calorie, high-fiber multigrain	13.6	12.7	0.9
Reduced-calorie, high-fiber white	12.8	12.3	0.5
Rye	8.3	6.8	1.5
White	1.9	1.3	0.6
Whole wheat	8.1	7.0	1.1

[a] Adapted from (11).

TABLE 3-2. Typical White Bread Formula

Ingredient	Percent Flour Basis
Flour	100
Water	64
Yeast	2.5
Salt	2.0
Sugar	8.0
Shortening	2.75
Yeast food	0.50
Nonfat dry milk	2.0
Mono- and diglycerides	0.5

EFFECTS OF HIGH-FIBER INGREDIENTS ON BREAD

High-fiber ingredients affect the formulation and processing of bread to some extent. These effects are discussed below.

Water absorption of the dough. High-fiber ingredients, which can be added at either the sponge stage or the dough-mixing stage, increase the water-absorption properties of the dough. The extent of this effect depends on the amount and type of fiber(s) used. The water-binding properties of the fiber can be an indication of the likely dough absorption changes (7). Farinograph measurements have shown that, as the concentration of fiber increases (the fibers used were cellulose and oat, apple, and pea fibers), the water absorption increases (8). Additional water is usually necessary in the formulation to adequately hydrate the gluten as well as the added fiber.

Presoaking the fiber before addition to the sponge or dough aids in the mixing process and may decrease the crumbliness of the final bread (3,6,9). The structures of sugar beet fiber in a presoaked state as well as a dry state are shown in Figure 3-1. Presoaking permits expansion of the fiber and preferential hydration because there are no other ingredients, such as gluten or starch, that compete for the water. The amount of additional water needed is not easy to determine, and experiments with mixing time (see below), baking conditions (such as time and temperature), loaf volume, and finished moisture can help in determining the additional amount of water necessary (10).

Mixing time. In general, the addition of high-fiber ingredients requires an increase in the mixing time of the dough. The increase is necessary to ensure complete hydration of the dough as well as the formation of gluten. Formation of the gluten matrix is hindered because the fiber molecules obstruct the flour proteins from coming together and combining to form gluten. Use of a strong-gluten (i.e., high-protein) flour can help, but usually the addition of vital wheat gluten is necessary to increase the proportion of protein molecules that can form gluten.

Gluten-enhancing agents such as methylcellulose (MC), dough strengtheners, and/or oxidizing agents can also be used. MC increases

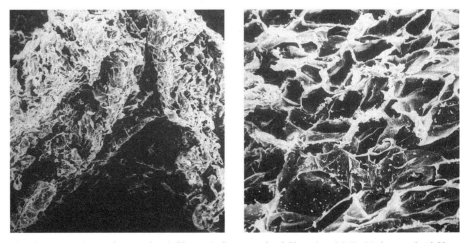

Fig. 3-1. Structure of sugar beet fibers. Left, unsoaked fiber (× ~300). Right, soaked fiber (× ~300). (Courtesy Fibrex/Danisco Sugar, Sweden)

the dough viscosity during baking. Other gums such as guar, locust bean, or carboxymethylcellulose (CMC) can also be helpful for increasing dough viscosity. The gas cells that expand during fermentation are stabilized by the interfacial activity of the MC (11). MC also reversibly gels with heat and can therefore help to set the crumb structure during baking (6,11). Dough strengtheners are surfactants that increase the ability of the wheat proteins to interact with one another to form gluten (1). As also mentioned above, oxidizing agents such as ascorbic acid or bromate can increase the ability of the wheat proteins to form gluten.

In addition, high-fiber ingredients in doughs generally result in decreased tolerance to overmixing (6–8,10,11). Experimentation with mixing time is helpful in understanding the effect of the amount and type of fiber on the final quality of the loaf.

Crumb grain and texture. The addition of high-fiber ingredients may negatively affect the crumb grain. This results mainly from the insufficient formation of a gluten network. The use of strong gluten flours, the addition of vital wheat gluten, or the use of gluten-enhancing agents such as MC, dough strengtheners, or oxidizing agents helps to bring about uniform porosity of the crumb grain. The section above on mixing time discusses the mechanisms of these agents. If wheat bran is used, prefermentation of the bran by yeast or yeast and lactic acid bacteria or the use of commercial baking enzymes has also been shown to improve the crumb structure.

Poor mouthfeel (i.e., grittiness) has been noted in products containing high-fiber ingredients. Choosing the appropriate particle size and/or length of fiber can control this phenomenon. Reduction of the particle size of wheat bran was reported to improve the crumb structure and mouthfeel of high-fiber wheat bread. Due to their length, fibers greater than 150 μm long have caused problems with dough development and with slicing of the final product (5). However, if these fibers are used at low levels (less than 2%), they can improve the dough and crumb strength (5). In general, as the length of the fiber increases, the grittiness or poor mouthfeel increases. However, the effect on mouthfeel varies depending on the type of fiber, concentration, and processing treatments used during the manufacture of that ingredient (12).

The use of high-fiber ingredients has also been related to positive effects on the texture of breads and related products. The addition of fibers can enhance the softness of the crumb because the fibers are able to bind water and hold it through the baking process. Fibers that are high in soluble fiber (for example, apple, sugar beet, prune, or date fibers, or psyllium) can positively influence the softness of the crumb by helping to retain moisture and by increasing the perception of crumb moistness. The addition of low levels (0.5%) of arabinogalactans can increase the crumb fineness and improve the cell shape of white pan bread (13). The use of inulin in bread can result in a uniform, finely grained crumb structure.

Color. Because high-fiber ingredients can contain colors that were present in the source from which they were derived, the color may be evident in the final product. This may be a desirable effect for breads such as whole wheat or multigrain. However, the developer of a white pan bread may want the product to remain white. Some high-fiber ingredients are naturally whiter than others (for example, resistant starch). However, for those that are not as white, many ingredient processors overcome the problem by bleaching the ingredient. This was discussed in Chapter 2.

Freshness and shelf-life. The freshness of bread products and the perception of their freshness are related to many factors. The main contributor to freshness perception is moisture content. The typical moisture content of breads can range, depending upon the final product, from about 20 to about 40%. As mentioned above, the addition of fibers can enhance the softness of the crumb, since many fibers can bind water and hold it through the baking process. Low levels of gums and soluble fibers such as sugar beet fibers or inulin can aid the moisture retention properties of both frozen doughs and final bread products, improving the shelf-life of these products. Fibers also help to inhibit moisture migration during frozen storage. In addition, high-fiber ingredients decrease ice crystal formation in frozen doughs, which increases their *freeze-thaw stability.*

Fibers can also help to minimize staling and crumb firming of bread products. The softness of the crumb is retained, and it has also been shown that the staling rate can be reduced.

Loaf volume. One of the most noticeable effects of the addition of high-fiber ingredients to breads is the reduction in the final volume of the product. The proportion of gluten is lower if the fiber source is added as a straight replacement of the flour. This is called dilution of the gluten. However, the dilution of gluten does not account for the total loaf volume decrease. The additional decrease is thought to result from a reduction in the dough's gas retention ability caused by the presence of the high-fiber ingredients (7). Figure 3-2 shows the effect of added cellulose, wheat bran, and oat hull fiber on the loaf volume of white pan bread. The addition of dough strengtheners, shortening, and nonfat dry milk has been found to increase the loaf volume when high-fiber ingredients are present in the formula. The use of low levels of soluble fibers (i.e., about 2%) also increases loaf volume. For example, the addition of psyllium fiber at levels of 2, 4, and 8% significantly increases the volume of the loaf as well the softness of the crumb (14).

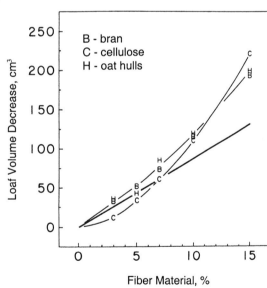

Fig. 3-2. Effects on loaf volume of replacing 3, 5, 7, 10, and 15% wheat flour by celluloses (C), wheat bran (B), or oat hulls (H). The values of C, B, and H are averages of seven, four, and two samples, respectively, and are compared with the theoretical loaf volume decrease (heavy straight line). (Reprinted, with permission, from [7])

Slicing operations. The addition of high-fiber ingredients can cause problems with slicing. Fibers with lengths greater than 150 µm have been found to cause difficulty in achieving a clean slice (5). The fibers can also cause rapid dulling of the blades, more so than with a typical white bread. In addition, slicing blades can become gummed because of the higher moisture content of the final product. Complete cooling of the bread is a critical step in decreasing this problem (6). The use of emulsifiers such as SSL or ethoxylated monoglycerides can help to reduce problems with the slicing blades becoming dull or gummed.

Cookies

High-fiber ingredients can be used in cookie formulations, and typically their purpose is to increase the TDF of the product. The dietary fiber contents of several varieties of cookies are given in Table 3-3. TDF levels of 4–5 g per cookie can be achieved (6). Reduced-fat cookies can also be made with these ingredients because many high-fiber ingredients also have fat-mimicking properties. There is a wide variety of cookie formulations, and the affect that high-fiber ingredients have on the final product varies with the formula type. For standard comparisons, fiber is used as a replacement for flour in a sugar snap cookie formula, and the results are compared with cookies made according to the control formula. A typical control formulation for a sugar snap cookie is shown in Table 3-4. Levels of added fiber can range from 0 to 30%. The effects of high-fiber ingredients in sugar snap cookie formulations are discussed below.

COOKIE SPREAD

The amount that the cookie dough spreads during baking is a quality measurement used in cookie baking tests. In general, a large spread is desirable in the manufacture of traditional cookies. The use of high-fiber ingredients with a high insoluble fiber content (cellulose, wheat bran, etc.) as well as more common cereal fiber sources (oat bran, soy fiber, etc.) decreases cookie spread (15–21). The decrease in spread results from the water-binding properties of the fibers. Figure 3-3 shows the effect of various fibers on the spread of a crisp sugar cookie.

TABLE 3-3. Typical Dietary Fiber Content (%) of Cookies[a]

| Type | Dietary Fiber | | |
	Total	Insoluble	Soluble
Butter	2.4	1.6	0.8
Chocolate chip	2.6	1.9	0.7
Fig bar	4.6	4.0	0.6
Ginger snap	1.8	1.2	0.6
Oatmeal	2.6	1.5	1.1
Peanut butter	1.8	1.3	0.5
Shortbread	1.8	0.9	0.9
Sugar	1.1	0.7	0.4
Vanilla wafer	1.5	0.7	0.8

[a] Adapted from (11).

TABLE 3-4. Typical Sugar Snap Cookie Formula

Ingredient	Percent	Percent Flour Basis
Soft wheat flour	45.4	100
Granulated white sugar	22.7	50
Shortening	20.4	45
Nonfat dry milk	2.3	5.0
Salt	0.5	1.0
Baking soda	0.4	0.8
Baking powder	0.7	1.5
Water	7.7	17.0

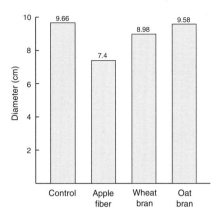

Fig. 3-3. Effect of fibers on cookie spread. Values shown are at a 12% substitution level of fiber for flour in a crisp sugar cookie formula. (Adapted from [22])

Hemicellulose components correlate most strongly with a decrease in cookie spread compared with other fiber components such as lignin (18). Hemicelluloses have a high water-binding capacity. As the amount of hemicelluloses in a fiber source increases, the cookie spread decreases (18). The addition of 1–2% lecithin improves cookie spread in the presence of high-fiber ingredients (17). Increasing the fat, sugar, and/or water level of the formula can also increase the spread. Also, not all fibers decrease the spread of the cookie. Highly soluble fibers such as fructooligosaccharides and inulin can help to increase it. Studies with the soluble fiber arabinogalactan have shown that use of 1, 2, and 5% of that fiber in a sugar snap cookie formula causes an increase in the cookie spread (13).

TENDERNESS AND CRISPNESS

The addition of high-fiber ingredients may cause an increase in the tenderness of the cookie crumb. This also corresponds with a decrease in cookie crispness but can vary depending on the fiber source (15–21). The increased tenderness can be attributed to the water-binding properties of high-fiber ingredients. Crispness can be increased by increasing the amount of crystallizable sugars such as sucrose in the formula (22). Trials with different baking times can also help to reduce the total moisture content of the cookie, but care must be taken to ensure that the product does not become too dry, brittle, or hard. Some fiber sources may also produce a powdery or gritty sensation. Since there are many different parameters of high-fiber ingredients that can influence these effects, experimentation with different particle sizes, fiber lengths, or fiber sources can help the user to determine the optimal ingredient parameters for a quality cookie.

TOP GRAIN AND SURFACE CRACKING

In general, the addition of high-fiber ingredients results in a poorer top grain appearance of the cookie. A desirable standard sugar-snap cookie has shallow, narrow crevices. Because the fibers absorb water, these cracks are usually not evident in high-fiber cookies. Increasing the amount of crystallizable sugars can help, but often a decrease in the amount of the high-fiber ingredient produces a more desirable top grain appearance (15–21).

COLOR

The color of the final cookie depends on the formula used (for instance, peanut butter cookies are darker than sugar cookies). For sugar-type cookies, where dark colors are not preferred, bleached fibers can be used to provide the desired effect.

FLAVOR

Some fibers can impart off-flavor to the final cookie product. Different fiber sources can be tried, or spices and flavors such as cinnamon, nutmeg, or vanilla can be used to mask the off-notes. Nutty flavors can also be added to a cookie product through the use of high-fiber ingredients that have been roasted or toasted.

Cakes, Muffins, and Other Batter Formulations

Incorporating high-fiber ingredients into cake, muffin, and other batter-type formulations such as pancakes and waffles is less challenging because these formulations contain more water than bread and cookie formulations. Hydrating both the flour and the fiber is less a problem than in breads because more water can be added to the batter to ensure complete hydration while controlling viscosity and having minimal impact on the final product. In general, high-fiber ingredients may be added to products such as cakes and muffins to raise the fiber content and/or reduce the fat content. As in the case of bread, other reasons for using high-fiber ingredients include improving moistness retention and freshness perception.

However, some problems can be encountered when using high-fiber ingredients in cake and related products at higher levels. For example, the use of high-fiber ingredients at levels greater than 40–50% of the formula can cause a decrease in the product volume and give poor mouthfeel characteristics (23,24). Muffins typically contain higher amounts of fiber. The typical fiber composition of various muffins is shown in Table 3-5.

When used at low levels, high-fiber ingredients can be beneficial to cakes and related products, and many different high-fiber ingredients can be successfully used in such formulations. Cellulose and cellulose derivatives are among the commonly known ingredients used in these applications. Early studies reported that the use of CMC improved the mouthfeel and shelf life of white layer cakes (25). CMC can be used at low levels (0.1–0.5%) to improve aeration and crumb quality (26). High-fiber ingredients used at low levels in cakes and related products increase crumb quality (i.e., uniformity, volume, tenderness, and moistness perception), act as suspension agents, and increase shelf life. These factors are further discussed below.

CRUMB QUALITY

High-fiber ingredients can increase the uniformity of the cellular structure of the crumb by acting as structural agents around

TABLE 3-5. Dietary Fiber Content (%) of Various Muffins

Type	Dietary Fiber		
	Total	Insoluble	Soluble
Blueberry	3.6	3.1	0.5
Bran-raisin	6.3	4.9	1.4
Oat bran	7.5	5.0	2.5
Plain	1.5	1.0	1.5
Wheat bran	3.3	2.5	0.8

the air cells of the product (6,12,27). Depending on the fiber type, typical substitution levels of fiber for flour can range from 0.5 to 10% with positive results. The fibers are able to reinforce the structure and allow for increased, more uniform expansion. This also results in higher volume, which in turn increases the yield of the product. The increased structural support can also benefit cake products by making them better able to withstand frosting loads. High-fiber ingredients can decrease the amount of shrinkage of the product upon cooling (6,12,27). They can also significantly improve crumb tenderness (6,12,27,28). This results from the ability of fibers to bind water, which also causes an increase in the perceived moistness of the crumb.

SUSPENSION AGENTS

The fibers in high-fiber ingredients form networks, reducing the ability of solid particles to settle out of a batter. In addition, they can increase the viscosity of the batter, which slows the particles' movement within it. Therefore, high-fiber ingredients are often used to suspend ingredients such as chocolate chips and nuts in cake, muffin, or pancake batters.

SHELF LIFE

The shelf life of baked goods such as cakes and related products can be improved by using high-fiber ingredients. The ability to bind water allows these ingredients to slow moisture migration from the product. This decreases the firming of the product and maintains the softness and moistness of the crumb (5,12,27,28). Also, fruit-based fiber products (such as date, prune, fig, and raisin powders and pastes) can extend shelf life by inhibiting the mold growth caused by the presence of naturally occurring acids and sorbitol (29–32).

Batters and Breadings

High-fiber ingredients are often used in the formulations for both batters and breadings, which provide coatings for foods that are usually deep fried, baked, or microwaved. Important characteristics of the formulations are that they remain on the product during processing and final consumer preparation and that they provide good texture (e.g., crispness, flakiness), good color, and low oil uptake during frying. High-fiber ingredients that contain a high proportion of insoluble fibers (e.g., cereal-based fibers such as corn or wheat bran) can be easily incorporated into breading formulas.

High-fiber ingredients such as gums, resistant starches, and cellulose derivatives provide several benefits to batter formulas (33). Unlike many starches, gums such as guar, xanthan, or CMC can provide viscosity without heating, which is useful for cold-batter systems. Also, these ingredients can suspend solids. MC and hydroxypropyl methylcellulose have the ability to gel with heat, which can cause them to form a barrier to oil, thus reducing oil pickup. Alginate, CMC, mycrocrystalline cellulose, and cellulose also reduce oil pickup by their ability to form a film. The water-binding ability of these ingredients aids in the adhesive and cohesive strength of the batter system. This also helps to provide freeze-thaw stability as well as to prevent moisture migration. In addition, these ingredients can provide crispness, texture, and lighter colors, all of which are positively associated with batters.

Other Baked Products

There are several other miscellaneous baked products into which high-fiber ingredients can be incorporated with beneficial results. These include low-moisture baked items such as crackers, tortilla or taco chips, and pretzels. The use of high-fiber ingredients containing insoluble fibers with longer lengths increases the strength of the product, which in turn reduces the amount of breakage. They can also make these products less crumbly and increase the snap, crispness, and crunch.

Extruded Products

Extruded products are of many different types, including pet foods, salty snacks, and ready-to-eat breakfast cereals. While the formulations for these product categories vary widely, the addition of high-fiber ingredients can have a similar affect on the formulation and end product, assuming that all other factors (other ingredients, use of steam, screw speed, etc.) remain constant. In these products, the basic structure of the final product strongly depends on the starch component. The starch in the formula, in the presence of water and the heat that is generated by precooking/preconditioning, shear frictional forces, and/or injected steam, gelatinizes to form the structural matrix. During extrusion, the water is subjected to high pressures and becomes superheated. When the product exits the die, the water becomes steam, expanding the starch and the product matrix.

In general, the addition of high-fiber ingredients that contain high proportions of either insoluble fibers or soluble fibers causes a decrease in the product's expansion when extruded, resulting in an increase in product density. The extruded product generally has smaller air cells and thicker cell walls. Also, because the fibers can reinforce the structure, extruded products with added fiber often are more resistant to breakage. The addition of 1–4% oat fiber has been found to reduce breakage in extruded snacks by up to 50% (34). At high levels, fibers can cause an increase in product breakage, since they begin to disrupt (rather than reinforce) the starch cell matrix, and the starch can no longer hold the structural matrix together. Resistant starches, on the other hand, have been found to increase product expansion. Products formulated with resistant starch are lighter in texture yet still have increased durability (35). In general, water-soluble fibers can also cause an increase in the ability of the final product to stick or pack into the teeth when eaten. Plant-based gums have different effects on the final extruded products, and experiments should be made with the desired formula to determine the effects with that formula (6).

The extrusion process has been studied for its effects on dietary fiber. In general, under mild or moderately severe conditions, extrusion does not cause a considerable change in the TDF of the product. However, some of the dietary fiber components are solubilized during extrusion (36). At high shear rates (severe extrusion conditions), the TDF of the extruded product can increase due to the formation of resistant starches (36).

Low-Fat Baked Goods

Many types of fat-replacing ingredients are available today. The major types can be placed into four categories: protein-based (i.e., microparticulated proteins), fat-based (i.e., emulsifiers, caprenin), synthetic (Olestra), and carbohydrate-based. The carbohydrate-based category covers a wide range, including maltodextrins, hydrocolloid gums, starches and modified starches, and cellulose. Many high-fiber ingredients function well as a source for fat replacement. Where labeling of ingredients is an issue, they allow the product developer to plainly label the food as containing ingredients that cause minimal consumer concern. In addition, high-fiber ingredients with high insoluble fiber content can be used to reduce the caloric content of the food. Calorie reduction can be significant, since the insoluble fiber contributes zero calories per gram; soluble fiber contributes four calories per gram; while the fat contributes nine calories per gram. High-fiber ingredients also can contribute health benefits by providing insoluble as well as soluble fiber to the diet. Often, blends of fibers from different sources can be used to create a fat-replacing system.

High-fiber ingredients exhibit many properties that enable them to function as fat replacers in baked goods. In general, they function as bulking agents or aeration agents, provide moistness/*lubricity*, provide creamy and fatlike textures, and extend the shelf life of reduced-fat baked goods. These properties are briefly defined below.

BULKING AGENTS

The formulation of reduced-calorie foods often involves replacing solids. Fibers can provide the bulk that was lost in removing the fat and/or sugars. Polydextrose and inulin can be used as bulking agents in reduced-fat or reduced-calorie baked goods.

AERATION

The *creaming* step is critical in the making of cakes as well as cookies. The entrapment of air is important in the formation of the air cells

Lubricity—A desirable slippery sensation in the mouth imparted by fats.

Creaming—The process of incorporating air into a fat matrix by rapidly mixing the fat with a crystalline sugar.

in cakes and also affects the texture of cookies. High-fiber ingredients can function as aeration agents in cakes and cookies. Some ingredients are also able to form gels with water, allowing them to replace the fat and incorporate the air into the gel system. Inulin is a gel-forming high-fiber ingredient that can be used in baked goods to aid in the aeration step.

MOISTNESS/LUBRICITY

Fat provides lubrication to baked goods and aids in the smooth mouthfeel of these products. This also creates a perceived moistness in the final baked good. The removal of fat often results in dry, crumbly baked goods with poor mouthfeel characteristics. Because fibers are able to bind water, they can enhance the mouthfeel of low-fat baked goods.

SHELF-LIFE EXTENSION

The extension of the shelf life of foods is related to the ability of high-fiber ingredients to bind water, allowing the product to retain its moistness.

Troubleshooting

BAKED GOODS—GENERAL		
Symptom	**Causes**	**Changes to Make**
Rapid drying and staling of product; limited shelf life	Inadequate water absorption or retention	Add low levels (typically less than 5%) of high-fiber ingredient to formulation.
Very low batter viscosity or sticky doughs[a]	Water level too high	Check calculations of water content. Be sure that water uptake of high-fiber ingredients is considered, and adjust free water addition accordingly.
	Too much high-fiber ingredient	Reduce high-fiber ingredient level. Try a lower-water-binding fiber or a fiber that has been processed for lower water-absorption properties.
Gritty texture	Incorrect particle size or fiber length of high-fiber ingredient	Experiment with both larger and smaller particle sizes and adjust ingredient requirements with supplier. Prehydrate high-fiber ingredient before addition to formula. Precoat high-fiber ingredient (with a fat source, etc.).
Off color (too dark)	Presence of pigments from high-fiber ingredients	Use high-fiber ingredients that are either bleached to remove pigments or are white (e.g., resistant starch).

BREADS AND RELATED YEAST-RAISED PRODUCTS		
Symptom	Causes	Changes to Make
Crumbly, dry crumb	Insufficient hydration of ingredients	Presoak high-fiber ingredients in water before adding to formula.
		Check calculations of water content. Be sure that water uptake of high-fiber ingredients is considered, and adjust free water addition accordingly.
		Reduce high-fiber ingredient level.
		Try a lower-water-binding fiber or a fiber that has been processed for lower water-absorption properties.
	Low water-binding capabilities of ingredients in formula	Add a high-fiber ingredient at a low level (typically less than 5%).
Low loaf volume, poor crumb grain	Insufficient gluten formation	Increase mixing time.
		Add agents to increase or enhance gluten formation such as: Vital wheat gluten, Dough strengtheners (SSL or ethoxylated monoglycerides), Oxidizing agents (ascorbate, potassium bromate, methylcellulose).
		Add commercial baking enzymes.
Off-flavors or odors	Natural flavor/odor of high-fiber ingredient	Work with supplier to remove flavor through processing.
		Try another high-fiber ingredient source.
		Check quality of incoming ingredients.
Off-color (darker than desired)	Presence of pigments from high-fiber ingredients	Use high-fiber ingredients that are either bleached to remove pigments or are white (e.g., resistant starch).
Poor slicing characteristics (blades dull easily or build gummy residue easily)	Presence of long fibers	Reduce fiber length.
		Cool product completely before slicing.
		Add emulsifier to formula.
SWEET GOODS—GENERAL		
Symptom	Causes	Changes to Make
Tough and/or dry crumb	Low water level in formula	Check calculations of water content. Be sure that water uptake of high-fiber ingredients is considered, and adjust free water addition accordingly.
	Insufficient hydration of ingredients	Reduce high-fiber ingredient level.
		Try a lower-water-binding fiber or a fiber that has been processed for lower water-absorption properties.
		Presoak high-fiber ingredients in water before adding to formula.
	No water-binding ingredients in formula	Add a high-fiber ingredient at a low level (typically less than 5%).

Excessive batter viscosity,[a] usually resulting in small, sticky, gummy crumb structure and/or high-density products	Too much high-fiber ingredient	Reduce high-fiber ingredient level. Experiment with other high-fiber ingredient sources.

CAKES, MUFFINS, AND RELATED PRODUCTS

Symptom	Causes	Changes to Make
Low volume	Little or no aeration during creaming step	Increase granulation size of sweetener. Add a high-fiber ingredient that improves aeration during creaming (e.g., CMC).
Collapsed structure	Starch gelatinization restricted due to competition for water by high-fiber ingredients	Check calculations of water content. Be sure that water uptake of high-fiber ingredients is considered, and adjust free water addition accordingly. Reduce high-fiber ingredient level. Try a lower-water-binding fiber or a fiber that has been processed for lower water-absorption properties. Presoak high-fiber ingredients in water before adding to formula.
Tough, dry crumb	Insufficient hydration of ingredients	Presoak high-fiber ingredients in water before adding to formula. Check calculations of water content. Be sure that water uptake of high-fiber ingredients is considered, and adjust free water addition accordingly. Reduce high-fiber ingredient level. Try a lower-water-binding fiber or a fiber that has been processed for lower water-absorption properties.
	Low water-binding capabilities of ingredients in formula	Add a high-fiber ingredient at a low level (typically less than 5%).
Very dark color	Presence of pigments from high-fiber ingredients	Use high-fiber ingredients that are either bleached to remove pigments or are white (e.g., resistant starch).
Coarse irregular crumb	Improper creaming	Increase creaming time. Increase granulation of sweetener used to aid incorporation of air during creaming. Add high-fiber ingredient that improves aeration during creaming (e.g., CMC).

COOKIES

Symptom	Causes	Changes to Make
Undesirable lack of surface cracking	High-fiber ingredient preferentially absorbs water, causing no separations in the dough matrix	Increase sweetener (sucrose) level. Decrease high-fiber ingredient level. Experiment with high-fiber ingredient with lower water-binding ability.

No snap; texture too soft	Little or no recrystallization of sugar due to presence of high-fiber ingredient network	Increase sucrose level. Decrease high-fiber ingredient level.
	Water bound by high-fiber ingredient	Experiment with lower-water-binding high-fiber ingredient. Increase baking time. Decrease liquids in formula.
Texture too hard	Insufficient hydration	Reduce high-fiber ingredient level. Try a lower-water-binding fiber or a fiber that has been processed for lower water-absorption properties. Presoak high-fiber ingredients in water before adding to formula. Increase fat content or add emulsifier such as lecithin.
	No water-binding ingredients in formula	Add a high-fiber ingredient at a low level (typically less than 5%).
Color too dark	Presence of high-fiber ingredient	Use high-fiber ingredients that are either bleached to remove pigments or are white (e.g., resistant starch).
Off-flavor	Natural flavor of high-fiber ingredient	Work with supplier to remove flavor through processing. Try another high-fiber ingredient source. Add masking flavor or spices. Check quality of incoming ingredients.

FROZEN BAKERY PRODUCTS

Symptom	Causes	Changes to Make
Poor freeze-thaw stability	Too little carbohydrate with high molecular weight	Add low levels (typically less than 5%) of high-fiber ingredient(s).

EXTRUDED PRODUCTS

Symptom	Causes	Changes to Make
Increased product breakage	Little starch network or structural matrix	Decrease level of high-fiber ingredient. Increase level of starch in formula.
	Starch network or structural matrix not reinforced	Add low levels (typically less than 5%) of high-fiber ingredient(s).
Increased toothpack	Highly dissolvable network or structural matrix	Decrease level of water-soluble fibers in formula. Increase insoluble:soluble fiber ratio.
Hard, dense product	Decreased expansion or puff	Increase level of starch. Increase moisture level of raw material before extrusion. Decrease high-fiber ingredient level. Prehydrate high-fiber ingredients before addition to extruder.

[a] Batter or dough viscosity can also be influenced by the type of flour used and the flour-to-sweetener ratio. Be sure that bread flour is used with yeast-raised products and cake flour with cakes and cookies. Also, ensure that the ratios of flour to sweetener and high-fiber ingredient to flour are not too high.

References

1. Stauffer, C. 1999. *Emulsifiers*. American Association of Cereal Chemists, St. Paul, MN.

2. Kulp, K. 1988. Bread industry and processes. Pages 371-406 in: *Wheat: Chemistry and Technology*, 3rd ed. Y. Pomeranz, Ed. American Association of Cereal Chemists, St. Paul, MN.

3. Vetter, J. L. 1988. Commercially available fiber ingredients and bulking agents. AIB Tech. Bull. 10(5):1-5.

4. Pechanek, U., Wutzel, H., and Pfannhauser, W. 1990. Dietary fibre enrichment, a sign of quality: Possibilities in bread. Page 337 in: *Dietary Fibre: Chemical and Biological Aspects*. D. A. T. Southgate, K. Waldron, I. T. Johnson, and G. R. Fenwick, Eds. The Royal Society of Chemistry, Norwich, England.

5. Hebeda, R. E., and Zobel, H. F. 1996. *Baked Goods Freshness—Technology, Evaluation, and Inhibition of Staling*. Marcel Dekker, New York.

6. Dreher, M. L. 1987. *Handbook of Dietary Fiber: An Applied Approach*. Marcel Dekker, New York.

7. Pomeranz, Y., Shogren, M. D., Finney, K. F., and Bechtel, D. B. 1977. Fiber in breadmaking—Effects on functional properties. Cereal Chem. 54:25-41.

8. Lang, C. E., Neufeld, K. J., and Walker, C. E. 1990. Effect of fiber on dough rheology. AIB Tech. Bull. 11(11):1-6.

9. Sosulski, F. W., and Wu, K. K. 1988. High-fiber breads containing pea hulls, wheat, corn, and wild oat brans. Cereal Chem. 65:186-191.

10. Stauffer, C. 1991. Fiber and baking. In: *Milling and Baking News*, Reference Source issue, 1990-1991. Sosland Publishing Co., Kansas City, MO.

11. Cho, S., Prosky, L., and Dreher, M. L. 1999. *Complex Carbohydrates in Foods*. Marcel Dekker, New York.

12. Kuntz, L. A. 1994. Fiber: From frustration to functionality. Food Product Design 3:91-108.

13. Strouts, B. 1997. Evaluation of arabinogalactan in bakery products. Research report. American Institute of Baking, Manhattan, KS.

14. Czuchajowska, Z., Paszczynska, B., and Pomeranz, Y. 1992. Functional properties of psyllium in wheat-based products. Cereal Chem. 69:516-520.

15. Vratania, D. L., and Zabik, M. E. 1978. Dietary fiber sources for baked products: Bran in sugar-snap cookies. J. Food Sci. 43:1590-1594.

16. Gorczyca, C. G., and Zabik, M. E. 1979. High-fiber sugar-snap cookies containing cellulose and coated cellulose products. Cereal Chem. 56:537-540.

17. DeFouw, C., Zabik, M. E., Uebersax, M. A., Aguilera, J. M., and Lusas, E. 1982. Effects of heat treatment and level of navy bean hulls in sugar-snap cookies. Cereal Chem. 59:245-248.

18. Jeltema, M. A., Zabik, M. E., and Thiel, L. J. 1983. Prediction of cookie quality from dietary fiber components. Cereal Chem. 60:227-230.

19. Sievert, D., Pomeranz, Y., and Abdelrahman, A. 1990. Functional properties of soy polysaccharides and wheat bran in soft wheat products. Cereal Chem. 67:10-13.

20. Artz, W. E., Warren, C. C., Mohring, A. E., and Willota, R. 1990. Incorporation of corn fiber into sugar snap cookies. Cereal Chem. 67:303-305.

21. Chen, H., Rubenthaler, G. L., Leung, H. K., and Baranowski, J. D. 1988. Chemical, physical, and baking properties of apple fiber compared with wheat and oat bran. Cereal Chem. 65:244-247.

22. Alexander, R. 1999. *Sweeteners: Nutritive*. American Association of Cereal Chemists, St. Paul, MN.

23. Fondroy, E. B., White, P. J., and Prusa, K. J. 1989. Physical and sensory evaluation of lean white cakes containing substituted fluffy cellulose. Cereal Chem. 66:402-405.
24. Jasberg, B. K., Gould, J. M., and Warner, K. 1989. High-fiber, non-caloric flour substitute for baked goods, alkaline peroxide treated lignocellulose in chocolate cake. Cereal Chem. 66:209-212.
25. Bayfield, E. G. 1962. Improving white layer cake quality by adding CMC. Baker's Dig. 36:50-54.
26. Zecher, D., and Van Coillie, R. 1992. Cellulose derivatives. Pages 40-65 in: *Thickening and Gelling Agents for Food.* A. Imeson, Ed. Chapman and Hall, New York.
27. Anonymous. 2000. Qualicel: Benefiting baked goods. Technical brochure QC008.1. Cellulose Filler Factory Corporation, Chestertown, MD.
28. Yue, P., and Waring S. 1998. Resistant starch in food applications. Cereal Foods World 43:690-695.
29. Sanders, S. W. 1989. Dates in bakery foods. AIB Tech. Bull. 11(6):1-6.
30. Bamford, R. 1990. Use of figs and fig products in bakery foods. AIB Tech. Bull. 12(10):1-6.
31. Sanders, S. W. 1990. Prunes in bakery products. AIB Tech. Bull. 12(3):1-6.
32. Fagrell, E. 1992. Raisin usage in baked goods. AIB Tech. Bull. 14(4):1-8.
33. Meyers, M. A. 1990. Functionality of hydrocolloids in batter coating systems. Pages 117-141 in: *Batters and Breadings in Food Processing.* K. Kulp and R. Loewe, Eds. American Association of Cereal Chemists, St. Paul, MN.
34. Anonymous. 1999. Opta Food Ingredients—Texture update: Opta oat fibers provide yield improvement. Tech. bull. Opta Food Ingredients, Bedford, MA.
35. Anonymous. 1998. CrystaLean—RTE expanded cereal. Opta Food Ingredients application bull. R981202. Opta Food Ingredients, Bedford, MA.
36. Asp, N., and Bjork, I. 1989. Nutritional properties of extruded foods. Pages 399-434 in: *Extrusion Cooking.* C. Mercier, P. Linko, and J. M. Harper, Eds. American Association of Cereal Chemists, St. Paul, MN.

Beverage and Dairy Applications

Beverages

While foods such as breads, breakfast cereals, fruits, and vegetables are commonly thought of as sources rich in fiber, beverages can also be sources for fiber in the diet. Nutritional beverages have made a significant impact on the market worldwide. Beverages formulated to improve the health of the consumer are very popular in Japan, Europe, and the United States. Teas, shakes or "smoothies," complete meal or meal-replacement diet drinks, and fruit beverages are just a few examples in which ingredients such as vitamins, herbs, minerals, and antioxidants, as well as fibers, are incorporated in order to deliver a more healthful beverage.

Although ingredients containing soluble fiber (e.g., pectin, gum arabic, and inulin) are more prevalent in beverage formulations due to their ability to easily disperse in water, insoluble fibers may also be used. However, manipulations in the processing of the high-fiber ingredient and/or formulation may be necessary. Therefore, for powdered drink mixes where the consumer is responsible for the final preparation by adding water or other liquid, insoluble fibers may not be the most desirable, or additional preparation instructions may be necessary.

ADJUSTMENTS FOR INSOLUBLE FIBERS

Some high-fiber ingredients containing high proportions of insoluble fibers may be organoleptically detectable and may even cause a gritty mouthfeel (1). Choosing a shorter fiber length and smaller particle size can minimize this effect. Also, changing the particle size of the fiber powder may also make it disperse more easily into the final formulation. The effect of particle size on properties such as the dispersibility and solubility of a high-fiber ingredient depends on many factors, which were discussed in Chapter 2.

Reduction in particle size may raise some other issues. The fibers themselves contain pores within their structure. Depending on the initial fiber structure, the additional grinding may cause a decrease in the pore volume and in the ability of the fiber to absorb water. The decrease in particle size of oat fibers causes a decrease in the water absorption of the powder due to the decrease of the pore volume of the product. Wheat and soy fibers have small internal pore volumes, and their water-absorbing properties are not highly affected by a reduction in particle size.

Ingredients that contain high proportions of insoluble fibers may also settle out of solution. This problem can be addressed by using soluble fibers to aid the suspension of the insoluble fibers. Also, allowing the insoluble fiber ingredient to completely hydrate (with more time, more mixing, etc.) can help in decreasing the amount of settling. The addition of sugars also helps to increase the density of the continuous phase of the mixture, thus increasing the stability.

EFFECTS OF HIGH-FIBER INGREDIENTS

Both soluble and insoluble fiber sources can be used in beverage formulations to increase the total dietary fiber (TDF) content, add mouthfeel/texture, stabilize the system/emulsion/foam, suspend solids, and influence flavors. These factors are discussed below.

Increase in TDF content. High-fiber ingredients are often used at low levels (i.e., about 0.1–0.2%) to significantly impact the solution viscosity (see Chapter 2) and act as bodying agents, affecting the mouthfeel and texture of the beverage. At this level of use, there is no impact on the labeling declaration for dietary fiber per serving according to the labeling regulations of the United States and most other countries. The levels needed to affect the label declaration depend highly on the final formula, since their density (i.e., the number of grams in a serving) in the formula varies depending on the ingredients. Typical levels of a high-fiber ingredient that are needed to raise the TDF content of the product can range from 1 to 20% of a beverage formula, depending on the fiber source. In the United States, declarations of TDF can range from about 2 to 8 g per 8-oz. serving.

Typically, high-fiber ingredients that have a minimal impact on solution viscosity are used for increasing TDF content. They are either minimally processed (i.e., extracted from the source) or modified so that they have minimal impact on other characteristics (e.g., ground to reduce particle size to reduce mouthfeel). Highly soluble low molecular weight fibers such as inulin and fructooligosaccharides affect solution viscosity minimally due to their small size. Some minimally processed fibers that are higher in molecular weight exhibit low viscosity levels even at higher concentrations because they tend to remain globular in solution and the polymer backbones do not extend themselves when hydrated, which is what causes an increase in the viscosity of the solution. These fibers include gum acacia (or gum arabic) and arabinogalactan. High-fiber ingredients can also be modified so that they do not affect viscosity and can then be used at levels that affect the TDF of the product while remaining in suspension. Partially hydrolyzed guar gum exhibits very low viscosities and has the ability to remain in solution.

Soy-based ingredients can be used in beverage applications both to increase the fiber content and to add protein. Soy-based beverages are becoming prevalent in the health-based beverage market (2,3).

Influence on mouthfeel/texture. High-fiber ingredients are commonly used to influence the mouthfeel and texture of beverages. They can affect these parameters both because of their physical presence in the solution and because of their ability to affect the solution viscosity. The effect of these ingredients on solution viscosity was reviewed in Chapter 2. They act as bodying agents, adding bulk to beverages such as shakes or blended beverages. However, fibers can also negatively influence the mouthfeel of a beverage by causing grittiness. This problem can be resolved by changing the particle size of the fiber. The size necessary for a reduction of the grittiness depends on the fiber type. In general, the smaller the particle size, the better, but some particles may still be detected at a particle size of about 10 µm. In addition, if the particle size of the fiber becomes too small, the physiological effect of the fiber (e.g., laxation) may decrease. It is best to experiment with various particle sizes of the specific fiber type to determine the level of detection for that fiber and the given formulation.

Stabilization of systems. Beverages can have several types of physical form, including emulsions or foams. These types of system are by nature unstable. Over time, they tend to reach a more stable state in which their phases (i.e., flavors, water, air) become separate. There are several means to increase the stability of the system so that it remains an emulsion or foam. In general, the smaller the emulsion droplet, or the foam air cell, the more stable the system. Water-soluble high-fiber ingredients can help to decrease the droplet or cell sizes by aiding mixing and increasing the incorporation of air during the aeration process. They can also help to decrease the interfacial activity between the two phases. In addition, high-fiber ingredients cause an increase in the viscosity of the system, which slows the coalescence of the droplets, thus increasing the stability of the system.

Suspension of solids. High-fiber ingredients can form a matrix within the beverage that helps to suspend particles within the beverage system. The amount of fiber needed depends on both the size of the particulate or solid and the type of fiber. Insoluble fibers, in general, tend to settle out of solution. Soluble fibers such as gum arabic, arabinogalactan, or partially hydrolyzed guar gum can be used to help keep insoluble fibers such as cellulose suspended in the beverage.

Influence on flavors. The addition of high-fiber ingredients to a beverage formula can often enhance its flavor. The use of roasted fibers, such as a roasted corn bran, can add nutty flavors to beverages such as cappuccino formulations. Also, because the high-fiber ingredient may cause an increase in the viscosity of the beverage, the time that the beverage resides on the tongue can be extended, and the flavors may have more opportunity for impact.

However, because fibers themselves have flavors, may interact with a flavor, or may dilute the flavor, they have the potential to mask or decrease the flavor of the beverage product. Inulin and fructooligosaccharides impart some sweetness and have been used to help round the flavor of aspartame in beverage formulations. Partially hydrolyzed guar gum has been noted to mute top notes of flavors in beverages (4). If the fiber decreases the flavor, addition of or increases in the amount of flavoring agent may be necessary.

Some high-fiber ingredients may also cause off-flavors in the product due to their own inherent flavor. For example, cereal fibers can cause raw or haylike flavors, while soy fibers can add a beany note to the beverage. Processing treatments of the fiber ingredients, such as roasting, can reduce these off-flavor notes. Trials with different high-fiber ingredients may be necessary, or masking agents (such as flavors) may be needed.

CHOOSING HIGH-FIBER INGREDIENTS

Several matters must be considered when choosing high-fiber ingredients for a beverage formulation. Knowing the requirements of the final product is necessary in order to clarify which fiber sources would be most likely candidates for the formulation. Using the topics discussed in the preceding section as requirement criteria can help. For example, if the target beverage is a low-viscosity, high-fiber beverage, one would not choose guar gum as a main high-fiber ingredient, since it can build high viscosity at very low concentrations. Suggested high-fiber ingredients that can meet some basic requirements for various beverage applications are shown in Table 4-1. In some applications, the high-fiber ingredient can also fulfill several needs, such as suspending solids, adding fiber, and providing mouthfeel.

A systems approach may be useful in developing the formulation. Since cost can be a factor in choosing high-fiber ingredients, one can increase the fiber level with lower-cost fibers, while using low levels of the more costly fibers that build viscosity or impact mouthfeel. Also, a systems approach may be necessary to add an insoluble fiber while using another more-soluble fiber to keep it in suspension.

TABLE 4-1. Suggestions for Use of High-Fiber Ingredients in Beverage Applications

Beverage Requirement		Processing Requirement
Low Viscosity, High Fiber	High Viscosity, Low Fiber	To Build Viscosity, Add Fiber[a]
Arabinogalactan	Guar gum	Cereal-based fibers
Gum arabic	Tragacanth gum	Pectin
Partially hydrolyzed guar gum	Konjac flour	Sugar beet fiber
Inulin		Cellulose
Fructooligosaccharides		Modified celluloses
		Inulin
		Psyllium
		Pea fiber
		Apple fiber
		Prune, date, raisin, and fig fiber
		Polydextrose

[a] Granulation may influence functional properties. See Chapter 3 for discussion.

The gelation characteristics of soluble fibers should also be considered when formulating a beverage. These fibers can provide desirable effects such as providing a creamy mouthfeel for dairy beverages or yogurt drinks, but they can also gel the product to the extent that it is no longer pourable. Experiments with both the type and level of fiber are often necessary to determine these effects, especially since the ingredients of the given formula (e.g., sugars, minerals) can also play a role. For example, high-methoxy pectin, alginate, gellan, and iota-carrageenan can gel in the presence of calcium ions and may form a gel in a dairy beverage formulation. The gelation characteristics of the soluble fiber sources can be found in Chapter 2.

The pH of the final beverage product also has a significant impact on the choice of the high-fiber ingredients. Different high-fiber ingredients can react differently under the same pH conditions, so it is important to understand how the pH affects the specific fiber used. In general, the insoluble fiber types (i.e., cereal-based fibers and cellulose) are stable over a wide pH range. They do not hydrolyze at the low pH levels typically found in beverage-type applications. Fruit-based fibers (prune, fig, apple, etc.) are also generally stable under these conditions, but due to their acidic nature, they can also influence the pH of the system. Water-soluble fiber types generally can function within the pH spectrum found in beverage applications, but they usually have a pH range at which they are most effective.

Some soluble fibers do cause certain pH problems in beverage applications. For example, at pH <3, carboxymethylcellulose (CMC) can precipitate out of solution; it is most stable at a pH range of 7–9 (5). Inulin and fructooligosaccharides can hydrolyze at pH <4. Storage time and temperature can play a role in determining the amount of hydrolysis. Above pH 3.7, minimum hydrolysis of inulin occurs over a six-month time frame, while in a concentrated fruit beverage at pH 3.2, studies have shown ~20% hydrolysis of inulin at 20°C. Konjac flour is able to form a strong gel in alkaline conditions and can create a very viscous beverage in the absence of alkali, depending on the concentration.

Incorporation of the high-fiber ingredient into the formulation may require some experimentation. Powders with small particle sizes can tend to form "fish eyes" when added to liquids due to their poor wettability. Adding the ingredient slowly at a high shear level can aid in dispersing the ingredient into the formulation. However, fibers can cause an increase in foaming when blended at high shear rates. Decreasing the speed of blending reduces this effect, and premixing the fiber with the other dry solids and then dispersing in water also helps. High-fiber ingredients can also be agglomerated to aid dispersion or coagglomerated with other highly water-soluble ingredients to increase their wettability.

In addition, certain high-fiber ingredients have been modified to meet the needs of beverage formulations. For example, oat β-glucan ingredients have been developed from hydrolyzed oat flour to be used as a soluble fiber source in beverages (6,7). An oat-based ingredient containing high levels of β-glucan can be used at levels of 0.25% to add a fiber source to iced teas, juices, and other beverages while having minimal impact on viscosity (6). Other oat-based high-fiber ingredients have been developed to add sweetness to beverages by enzymatically hydrolyzing the oat starch present (7). Some of these ingredients can affect solution viscosities when used at levels greater than 1%. They are an unusual fiber source because they are derived from a cereal source and yet can be easily added to beverage formulations due to their modification.

Dairy Applications

High-fiber ingredients are found in some applications in dairy products such as cheese, yogurt, ice cream, and their related products. Most of these applications have involved the use of water-soluble fibers for their water-binding properties as well as their low detectability in the product itself. Insoluble fibers can also be used in limited applications. Interest in creating high-fiber dairy products exists as a means of marketing a healthier product by reducing fat and cholesterol and providing a health benefit in addition to calcium.

CHEESE

Typically, high-fiber ingredients are not found in formulations for traditional hard cheeses. However, the use of high-fiber ingredients as processing aids has found some use in cheese production. For example, CMC has been found to improve the output, texture, and body of cheese by enhancing the precipitation of whey proteins during fermentation (8). Insoluble fibers such as cellulose and oat fibers can be used as anti-caking agents for shredded cheeses. Dusting these ingredients onto the shredded cheese minimizes the formation of clumps in the final shredded product. Also, high-fiber ingredients have been used to formulate some processed cheeses. Wheat fiber has been shown to improve texture, improve storage stability, reduce *syneresis*, and enhance the melting properties of processed cheeses with no negative impact on the sensory quality of the cheese (9).

In formulating reduced-fat or nonfat cheeses and cheese spreads, fat-replacing ingredients are often necessary to aid in mouthfeel, stretch, and melting properties. Water-soluble fibers can be used at low levels to enhance the viscosity development, texture, smoothness, and creaminess of these products. Guar gum and other water-soluble fibers such as pectin and inulin have been used to replace the fat in cheese applications, helping to make the cheeses soft. Microcrystalline cellulose and carrageenan can be used to bind water in the formulation, which aids in decreasing the rubbery texture of reduced-fat cheese applications. These ingredients may need to be prehydrated or preblended with the other dry ingredients in order to be fully incorporated into the formula.

Syneresis—The separation of liquid from a gel; weeping.

YOGURT AND PUDDING PRODUCTS

The use of high-fiber ingredients in yogurt and pudding applications has been mainly for the functional benefits they impart to the product. Many water-soluble fibers such as CMC, locust bean gum, guar gum, alginates, carrageenans, pectin, and inulin, for example, are used as stabilizers. These ingredients have the ability to increase the product viscosity, inhibit syneresis, and improve textural attributes such as creaminess and can aid in forming the semisolid set structure desired in custard-style yogurts and viscous puddings. These ingredients are often added before the fermentation of the yogurt and may need to be preblended with other dry ingredients to aid in their dispersion into the fluid milk. Prehydration can also aid the incorporation of the high-fiber ingredients. They can also be added after the fermentation step, with preblending and prehydration as necessary.

High-fiber ingredients are also used in an effort to increase the TDF content of yogurt or pudding, which can add another benefit to a product that is already viewed by consumers as healthy. Incorporation of inulin into yogurt products has also been related to promotion of the growth of beneficial bifidobacteria in the colon (see Chapter 6). Soy and oat fibers in combination with gum arabic have been used to develop a high-fiber yogurt that exhibits no adverse taste or mouthfeel effects (10). Plain and Swiss-style fruited yogurts with TDF content ranging from 2.5 g up to 10 g per 8-oz serving can be achieved (10). However, research has shown that the addition of 1.32% oat fiber to a plain yogurt formula before fermentation can decrease the flavor quality of the yogurt, even though improving the body and texture of the product (11). Addition of insoluble fiber types can also accelerate the acidification rate of the yogurt fermentation (11,12).

As in beverage applications, the use of insoluble fibers such as corn bran, oat fiber, soy fiber, and rice bran can result in a gritty texture in the final yogurt (12). Of these fibers, oat fibers have been shown to give the best mouthfeel results (11,12). Experiments with particle sizes of the various fibers can help to minimize this effect. A patented process has also shown that the addition of milk to insoluble fibers with subsequent crushing can decrease the amount of grittiness associated with yogurts formulated with insoluble fibers (13).

Soy fibers can decrease product viscosity (12,14) due to the syneresis of the whey. Sugar beet fiber has also been found to cause syneresis and decreased viscosity in yogurt formulations at a level of 1.32% (12). However, lower levels of sugar beet fiber in yogurt can improve the product's consistency (15).

ICE CREAM AND FROZEN DESSERTS

The various types of ice cream formulations can range from hardpack to soft-serve products. As in the case with yogurts and puddings, the main use of high-fiber ingredients in an ice cream formulation is to stabilize the frozen emulsion and foam system. The same applies

Standard of identity—A legal standard, maintained by the FDA, that defines a food's minimum quality, required and permitted ingredients, and processing requirements, if any. Applies to a limited number of staple foods.

to other frozen dessert products such as frozen yogurts, ice milks, and sherbet formulations. Because of their properties, high-fiber ingredients can also be used to replace fat in these systems. Note, however, that, in the United States, terms such as "ice cream" have been defined and are based on the *standard of identity* of the product. This standard lists the requirements for the product, such as the required minimum of fat. Therefore, in reducing the fat content of an ice cream formulation, it is best to check the most recent and regional requirements for the product.

The type of high-fiber ingredient chosen as stabilizer depends on the given formula and type of product. In general, these ingredients are used at low levels (0–0.5%) in the formulation and function to provide smoothness and freeze-thaw stability, decrease sandiness and iciness, and decrease rapid melting. High-fiber ingredients affect these characteristics by their ability to bind water and/or form gels within the emulsion. They can also help to suspend particulates in the liquid emulsion before freezing. The more water and less fat in the formulation, the more difficult the product is to stabilize. The water tends to form larger ice crystals, causing icy textures and decreased creaminess. Such formulations usually require a more efficient stabilization system and may require the use of several types of high-fiber ingredients. Common stabilizers used in ice cream formulations include locust bean gum, guar gum, CMC, microcrystalline cellulose, alginate, carrageenan, and xanthan gum. Guar gum is often used since it is soluble in cold water, as is carrageenan, which interacts with the milk proteins and therefore prevents wheying off (i.e., separation) of the mix. Inulin has also shown the ability to replace 100% of the fat in an ice cream formulation while maintaining the product's smoothness and creaminess as well as inhibiting ice crystal growth during storage (16).

Insoluble fibers are not typically added to ice cream formulations due to their ability to cause a gritty mouthfeel. However, oats have recently been used as a main ingredient in producing a soft-serve frozen dairy dessert (17). The product ingredients consist of water, oats, flavor, and color. The particle size of the oat product was found to be key in producing a frozen product with a creamy, smooth mouthfeel. The product derives its sweetness from hydrolysis of the starch present in the oats. There is 1 g of TDF per 88-g serving of product.

Troubleshooting

BEVERAGES		
Symptom	**Causes**	**Changes to Make**
Lacks body and/or mouthfeel	Low viscosity or solids content	Add high-fiber ingredient to add mouthfeel.
Off-flavor/odor	Flavor from high-fiber ingredient	Add other flavors to mask. Try other high-fiber ingredient sources.
	Microbial or yeast growth	Check quality of incoming ingredients.

Low sweetness or flavor level	High-fiber ingredient masking sweetness or other flavor	Check processing, storage, and pH conditions against stability conditions of sweetener used. Increase sweetener/flavor level. Add alternative sweetening agent.
Gritty mouthfeel	Detectable particle size (fiber length) of high-fiber ingredient(s)	Decrease particle size of high-fiber ingredients.
	Insufficient viscosity of formulation	Increase viscosity of formulation.
Caking	Improper granulation of high-fiber ingredient	Increase granulation size of ingredients. Use anticaking agents. Store ingredient in dry environment.
Powder mix not homogeneous	Settling of large particles	Decrease granulation size of ingredients. Agglomerate mix to uniform particle size.
Poor dispersion into solution; formation of "fish eyes"	Poor particle wettability	Experiment with granulation size of ingredients. Agglomerate product.
Sedimentation, settling of ingredients	Poor suspendability of high-fiber ingredients	Add suspending agent such as water-soluble fiber (e.g., gum acacia, xanthan gum). Experiment with particle size of fiber source (typically decrease particle size).
Too much mouth cling	Component interaction	Experiment with particle size of fiber source (typically decrease particle size). Experiment with type of high-fiber ingredient.
Astringency; mouth drying	Component interaction	Experiment with type of high-fiber ingredient.
	Incorrect pH level	Check/adjust pH if possible.

CHEESE, PROCESSED CHEESE, SPREADS

Symptom	Causes	Changes to Make
Clumping of shredded cheeses	Ingredients adhering to each other	Add insoluble, small-particle high-fiber ingredient such as cellulose, oat fiber, or apple fiber.
Poor melt, stretch; rubbery texture; syneresis of reduced-fat cheese	Removal or reduction of fat content	Add high-fiber ingredient to simulate fat through water-binding properties.

YOGURTS, PUDDINGS

Symptom	Causes	Changes to Make
Low sweetness or flavor level	High-fiber ingredient masking sweetness or flavor	Check processing, storage, and pH conditions against stability conditions of sweetener used. Increase sweetener or flavor level. Add alternative sweetening agent.
Lack of body/texture	Low solids content	Add high-fiber ingredient, such as plant-derived gums.
Stringy texture	Lumpiness due to nonuniform particle distribution	Blend dry ingredients thoroughly before dispersion. Experiment with type of high-fiber ingredient.
Poor stability; syneresis	Poor water-holding ability	Add or increase high-fiber ingredients. Experiment with fiber type.
Gritty mouthfeel	Detectable particle size (fiber length) of high-fiber ingredient(s)	Decrease particle size of high-fiber ingredients. Experiment with fiber type.

ICE CREAM, FROZEN DESSERTS		
Symptom	**Causes**	**Changes to Make**
Too soft; icy; weak body	Low solids content	Add or increase level of high-fiber ingredients.
	Insufficient stabilizer	Add or increase level of stabilizer.
Coarse texture	Presence of large ice crystals	Increase level of stabilizer or of high-fiber ingredients.
Chewy or gummy texture	Excessive moisture binding by ingredients	Decrease level of stabilizer or high-fiber ingredients.
Gritty texture	Presence of high-fiber ingredients with large particle size	Decrease particle size of high-fiber ingredients. Experiment with other fiber sources. Decrease level of stabilizer or high-fiber ingredients.
Crumbly body; fluffy texture	High amount of air incorporation into formula (i.e., high overrun)	Increase level of stabilizer or high-fiber ingredients.

References

1. Hegenbart, S. 1995. Using fiber in beverages. Food Product Design 5(3):68-78.
2. Anonymous. 1997. Grains to fortifiers and nutraceuticals. Prepared Foods 166(9):65-71.
3. Glenn, C. 2000. Formulating products with soy. Internet resource: Food Explorer, Tech Tutorial (www.foodexplorer.com).
4. Greenberg, N. A., and Sellman, D. 1998. Partially hydrolyzed gum as a source of fiber. Cereal Foods World 43:703-707.
5. Zecher, D., and Van Coillie, R. 1992. Cellulose derivatives. Pages 40-65 in: Thickening and Gelling Agents for Food. A. Imeson, Ed. Chapman and Hall, New York.
6. Portnoy Kelley, K. 1993. Hey Rocky! Watch me pull a healthy drink outta my hat. Bev. Ind. 64(5):25-27.
7. LaBell, F. 1998. A sweet approach to added fiber. Prepared Foods 167(11):88.
8. Hansen, P. M. T., Hildago, J., and Gould, I. A. 1971. Reclamation of whey protein with carboxymethylcellulose. J. Dairy Sci. 54:830-834.
9. Anonymous. 1998. Wheat fibre—A beneficial ingredient for processed cheese. Eur. Dairy Mag. 9(4):35-36.
10. Hoyda, D. L. Streiff, P. J., and Epstein, E. 1990. Method of making fiber enriched yogurt. U.S. patent 4,971,810.
11. Fernandez-Garcia, E., McGregor, J. U., and Traylor, S. 1998. The addition of oat fiber and natural sweeteners in the manufacture of plain yogurt. J. Dairy Sci. 81:655-663.
12. Fernandez-Garcia, E., and McGregor, J. U. 1997. Fortification of sweetened plain yogurt with insoluble dietary fiber. Z Lebensm. Untersuch. Forschung. 204:433-437.
13. Anonymous. 1990. Yogurt containing water insoluble dietary fiber. Japanese patent JP4141045A.
14. Radwan, H. M. 1996. Production and evaluation of soymilk fortified yogurt. Ann. Agric. Sci. (Cairo) 41(1):281-292.
15. Saldami, I., and Babacan, S. 1996. Addition of dietary fibre to yoghurt. Gida 21:185-191.
16. Wouters, R. 1998. Nice—But not naughty. Dairy Foods 99(7):25-26.
17. Mannie, E. 1998. Tapping the power of enzymes. Prepared Foods 167(5): 123-126.

Other Applications

Jams, Jellies, and Preserves

The gelling of fruit-based mixtures produces jams, jellies, and preserves. Jams typically contain fruit pieces or crushed fruit; jellies are made with the juice extracted from the fruit; while preserves are generally made of the crushed, entire fruit. For simplification of this discussion, the term "jam" will be used to refer generally to this product category. The most widely used gelling agent in the production of jam is pectin. While pectin is a high-fiber ingredient, its use at low levels (typically less than 1%) in jam does not significantly contribute to the total dietary fiber (TDF) content of the product. The function of pectin is complex and can depend on many factors such as the type of pectin used, the pH and temperature, and the soluble solids (sugar) and calcium content of the formula.

Pectins of many varieties are available for use in making jam. The two types of pectins traditionally used are high-methoxy pectins and low-methoxy pectins (see Chapter 2). In general, the high-methoxy pectins gel under acidic conditions (pH levels of about 2.9–3.6), with a soluble solids range of about 60–80%. The several types of high-methoxy pectin available vary in their degree of esterification. In general, the greater the pectin's degree of esterification, the faster the setting time. High-methoxy pectins form gels that quickly become stable. Low-methoxy pectins require calcium salts, such as calcium citrate, for gelation. Since low-methoxy pectins require a lower soluble solids concentration (i.e., less dissolved sugars) than high-methoxy pectins, they are often used to make low-sugar jams. Gels formed using low-methoxy pectins are thermally reversible.

Certain processing procedures can aid in producing a high-quality final product. Pectins should be fully dispersed in the formula and should not be subjected to overcooking. The pH of the mixture should also be monitored since jams can exhibit syneresis over time if the pH of the system is too low. Pregelling is undesirable, and buffered pectins are available so that the pectin gels at the appropriate pH upon addition of acid to the formula. Once the formula is fully cooked, the hot, liquid suspension should be transferred immediately into the final product container. If the cooled product is transferred, a grainy product can result.

Other hydrocolloids can be used as the sole gelling agent or in addition to pectin to produce a jam-type product. Gums such as carrageenan and locust bean gum can replace solids and bulk in low-sugar jams and jellies. Gellan gum also can be used since it exhibits good stability in low-pH systems. The gelation characteristics as well as the textural attributes vary depending on the soluble solids content of the formulation.

Icings, Frostings, and Glazes

The high-fiber ingredients used in icing, frosting, and glaze applications typically are water-soluble fibers. These ingredients can bind water and enhance the adhesion of the system to the product (e.g., frosting to cake) because of their ability to enhance film-forming properties. Water-soluble fibers such as pectin, inulin, and gum arabic can also be used to replace fat in frosting-type applications by providing lubricity, viscosity, and texture. Also, the ability to bind water can help to decrease the migration of moisture from the frosting application to the baked product. Gum acacia is noted as a good emulsifier, while low-methoxy pectin and xanthan gum can be used in glaze-type applications because of their ability to form films. Sodium alginate and gum acacia can also help to reduce the tackiness of a frosting formulation, to keep it from adhering to the product wrapper. The use of hydrocolloids in frosting, glazes, and icings is reviewed elsewhere (1).

Confectionery

Confectionery products such as chocolate, soft confections, or hard candies are not typically high-fiber-containing foods. However, some confections containing high amounts of TDF have been developed. For example, a low-calorie confection containing microcrystalline cellulose and gum arabic at levels of 11–28% and 18–26%, respectively, has been patented (2). The confection also contains high-fructose corn syrup, condensed skim milk, and vegetable fat. According to the patent, the calorie content was reduced more than 55% with no loss of texture or flavor as compared to the high-calorie counterpart. In another patented soft confection application, guar gum, gum arabic, and pectin were used to increase the TDF content of a taffylike confection (3). Another patented soft confection also contained gum arabic (4). Gum arabic can be used at high levels in confectionery products because of its ability to add high levels of fiber without significantly affecting the formula's viscosity or the mouthfeel of the final product. It is also able to emulsify the other ingredients in the formulation, which can improve the texture and consistency of the product.

The use of high-fiber ingredients in various confections can also help to provide various functional benefits to these products. The ingredients provide gelation, viscosity, texture, lubricity, and mouthfeel and can add bulk solids when fats or sugars are removed. The use of high-fiber ingredients is discussed for several types of confections below.

CHOCOLATES

The general process for chocolate manufacturing involves the mixing of cocoa liquor, sweetener, and cocoa butter. This mixture is refined and then conched. Conching is the slow mixing and heating of the chocolate paste to reduce particle size and increase thickness and smoothness of the chocolate paste. Additional cocoa butter can also be added during the conching step. Dry conching refers to the process with no addition of cocoa butter, whereas wet conching involves the addition of cocoa butter during conching. Conching temperatures range from 40 to 82°C, depending on the desired end product (i.e., lower temperatures for milk chocolate, higher temperatures for dark chocolate). Conching is also responsible for the evaporation of volatiles and moisture as well as the development of flavors. In general, higher conching temperatures are preferred for flavor development and are used in the manufacture of dark chocolates.

Polydextrose can be used in reduced-sugar or sugar-free chocolate applications to replace solids content and can be used with higher conching temperatures (5,6). Initially, polydextrose could not be used in making chocolates or various other confections since the acidity levels caused by the polydextrose in these products caused inversion of sucrose. Forms of polydextrose that have low levels of residual acidity are now available for use in confections (7,8). The use of polydextrose in chocolate production has also been noted to enhance the flow properties of the chocolates during processing (6).

Other high-fiber ingredients can also be used in the manufacturing of chocolate and related products. High-fiber ingredients have been investigated in an attempt to replace cocoa butter in a chocolatelike product containing cocoa butter, sucrose, and flavor (9). The substitution of microcrystalline cellulose and guar gum for the cocoa butter was found to decrease the sweetness, flavor, and melting of the product as compared to the control. The amount of decrease in these three characteristics was proportional to the amount of substitution (the levels ranged from 5 to 20% replaced). There was also an increase in viscosity as well as increased perceived particle size with the cocoa butter replacement. Substitution with guar gum decreased the levels of sweetness, flavor, and melting to a greater extent than did substitution with microcrystalline cellulose.

Inulin has also been investigated as a replacement for sucrose and fat in chocolate products. A study in which inulin was used in a reduced-calorie formulation (5) found that dry conching alone was not acceptable since the chocolate mass became too viscous and the mass could not be heated over 70°C. Also, the final product was sandy in texture. When the chocolate mass formulated with inulin was subjected to a combination of dry and wet conching, the conching temperature could reach 80°C and the resulting chocolate product had significantly improved mouthfeel and melting properties. Additionally, inulin is commonly used in Europe to replace sugar in low-calorie and diabetic chocolate products.

Cocoa fiber from cocoa hulls can also be used to enhance the dietary fiber content of chocolates. One patent relates a process for producing a cocoa dietary fiber from cocoa powder. The product's suggested use is for dietary-fiber-enriched chocolate, dietary-fiber-enriched chocolate spreads, and candy (10).

SOFT CONFECTIONS

The category of soft confections is quite broad, encompassing confections such as taffy, caramel, nougats, fondants, chewing gums, and gummy-type candies. The use of high-fiber ingredients in this category (other than to achieve high fiber content, as described above) is limited to the use of gums and hydrocolloids for functional purposes. While gelatin has been a primary gelling agent in this segment, the use of pectin is also widespread in gummy confections and fruit leather-type products. Pectin helps to increase the remelt temperature, which also increases the stability during storage and shipping (11). High-methoxy pectin has been found to produce gels that are more fruity, tarter, and sweeter than gels formed using gelatin (12). Pectins also produce a clean bite or break. Typically, pectin and gelatin are used in combination in gummy-type confections. The amount of buffer, acid, gelatin, and pectin (as well as pectin type) all factor into the gelation of the system.

Gum arabic is another water-soluble high-fiber ingredient used in confectionery applications. It has been found to stabilize the sugar crust that enrobes liqueur-filled chocolates (13). Polydextrose can be used to replace solids in reduced-sugar soft confections such as caramels, gum drops, and taffy (7). Inulin has also been used in soft confections to enhance softness and increase the shelf life of the product.

HARD CANDIES

Because of their water-binding properties, water-soluble fibers are not widely used in hard-candy types of confections. Polydextrose can be used to replace solids, as a bulking agent, in sugar-free or reduced-sugar hard candies (8). Inulin has also been used in combination with isomalt to produce sugar-free hard confections. Other insoluble fibers typically interfere with the glass matrix formed in the hardening of molten sucrose, causing crystallization, graininess, and mouthfeel problems.

Meat, Poultry, Seafood, and Analog Products

This category contains a vast array of products, which include whole-muscle foods; restructured items such as sausages, links, and patties; and reduced-fat products. Increased understanding of the science behind these products has led to the development of many interrelated products that were once commonly thought of as made from beef. For example, salmon burgers, turkey hot dogs, and chicken sausages can be found in the marketplace today. Many types of protein sources can be used to manufacture these products. Beef, lamb, pork, chicken, turkey, fish, and shellfish are the major protein sources commonly used.

Many other ingredients are used in these products to create a desirable food that functions well for the consumer under various conditions (freeze-thaw cycles, grilling, frying, broiling, etc.). The governing agency in each country often stipulates the use levels and functions of these ingredients. For example, in the United States, strict requirements are placed on all meat and poultry ingredients used in restructured products. The ingredient must be approved, and the use level is stipulated by the USDA. Since these regulations can frequently change, it is best to check with the governing agency regarding any stipulations on the use of high-fiber ingredients in these formulations. Usage levels that impart functionality in products are typically fairly low (usually less than 3%) and vary depending on the high-fiber ingredient as well as the product requirements.

High-fiber ingredients can provide several types of functionalities depending on the product and the ingredient used. In formulations for restructured protein products such as patties, links, and sausages, their use is primarily as a binding agent. They can hold the proteins and other ingredients in the formulation by interacting with the proteins and water in the formula. Insoluble fibers can also add texture to these products, while soluble fibers (e.g., Konjac flour, inulin, alginate, carrageenan, pectin, curdlan, and gellan) are often used for their ability to form a gel that holds the ingredient matrix together. Because of the varying functional properties of high-fiber ingredients (see Chapter 2), a multi-ingredient systems approach is often used in formulating these products. The properties that these ingredients can influence are further discussed below.

PROPERTIES AFFECTED

Water binding. The ability of the high-fiber ingredient to bind water helps to maintain juiciness and lubricity. It also helps to increase the freeze-thaw stability and decrease a condition called "purge," the release of water from the product matrix, which results in a drier finished product. In low- or reduced-fat products, the ability of the high-fiber ingredient to bind any additional water in the formula becomes a necessary factor in the ability of the product to retain its desired shape and to have sliceability. In applications using ground beef fillings, high-fiber ingredients such as oat fiber help to reduce the amount of free water that can occur after frying (14). The binding of water also helps to improve the yield of the cooked final product.

Common high-fiber ingredients used to bind water include cereal fibers, cellulose, sugar beet fiber, and microcrystalline cellulose, as well as many plant-based gums. Carrageenans (at typical levels of 0.5–1.5%) are often used in formulating low-fat meat applications because of their ability to form complexes with meat proteins. Other water-soluble fibers such as locust bean gum, xanthan gum, inulin, and gellan gum can also be used.

Reduced weight loss and shrinkage. High-fiber ingredients also can help to reduce the weight loss of the product. The replacement of fat by these ingredients leads to less loss of the fat through dripping during finish processing such as broiling or frying. Because these ingredients also tend to hold water, as described above, less water is lost during these and other heating processes. The product also shrinks less because, although the muscle fibers still shrink upon heating, the high-fiber ingredients maintain their structural integrity.

Texturization. The use of high-fiber ingredients can add texture to restructured meat, poultry, vegetarian meat analogs, and seafood products. Most meat and poultry products already have a fibrous texture, so the use of these fiber-containing ingredients to help restructure the proteins can aid the final product's texture and mouthfeel. Their water-binding ability, as discussed above, allows many fibers to tenderize the product as well as to provide moistness.

In seafood products, the delicate texture of crab is often a factor affecting the final product formulation. Konjac flour can be used at low concentrations (typically 0.3–2%) to mimic this texture in products such as fish patties, surimi, and other imitation-crab products. It is also able to form a thermally stable gel under alkaline conditions that retains moisture and enhances the elasticity of the product. The stability of the gel improves with heat, which improves the overall final cooked quality of the product. This heat resistance of Konjac gels is a unique property that can be used for formulating products that need to retain moisture upon grilling, frying, or other intense heating. Because Konjac can form a white gel (under alkaline conditions or synergistically with starch, xanthan gum, or carrageenan), it can also be formed into small white particles and mixed into the formulation to resemble bits of fat in restructured reduced-fat meat products.

Pectin is a water-soluble fiber that can be used to form a brittle type of gel, which can help the product to have a clean bite as well as sliceability. Curdlan can also be used to form a heat-stable gel in many products. It has been shown to improve texture and physical properties such as elasticity and bite in meat-type gels (15).

While soy protein isolates are commonly used in reduced-fat or vegetarian analog meat products, soy protein concentrates, which contain about 25% dietary fiber, can also be used. The presence of soy fiber can help to mimic the fibrous texture associated with meat products such as hamburger patties. It also can help to emulsify the formulation, aiding in the homogeneity of restructured products or vegetarian analog products. Wheat fibers, rice bran, corn bran, cellulose gum, or sugar beet fibers can also be used to add texture (16). Oat fibers are widely used in meat applications to provide texture and bind moisture.

The use of some high-fiber ingredients may cause problems with mouthfeel and texture. Coarser fibers can cause poor texture and mouthfeel in the final product. For example, the use of 5–10% wheat bran or barley bran in low-fat beef sloppy-joe formulas was found to cause poor sensory qualities such as poor mouthfeel and poor juiciness (17).

FORMULATION CONSIDERATIONS

Two major factors need to be considered when formulating these types of products.

pH. The pH of the system strongly influences the choice of the high-fiber ingredient used. The pH must be considered because, if the protein reaches its *isoelectric point*, the ability of the protein to bind with other ingredients, such as a gum, would be affected. For example, the isoelectric point of meats ranges from pH 5.0 to 5.2. Carrageenan forms a complex with meat proteins below this pH level. If the pH of the formulation is 5.0–5.2 or above, the proper binding of the carrageenan to the meat proteins may not occur. Acidic conditions also may cause hydrolysis of gums. The pH of the system plays a role in gel forming also. For example, Konjac flour needs alkaline conditions (pH of about 9) in order to gel, while low-methoxy pectins require acidic conditions (pH 2.9–5.5). Unlike pectins, once alkaline conditions are achieved, the konjac flour gels remain stable at any pH level.

Dispersibility. The low level of water in these formulas makes it difficult for high-fiber ingredients to properly hydrate and disperse homogeneously throughout the system. In addition, the ingredients can form clumps, or dry spots in the product, if they are not added properly. Therefore, high-fiber ingredients often must be prehydrated before being added to the formula. Preblending with other dry ingredients in the formula may also be possible, depending on the type of formulation. For formulations where the formation of a gel is important, the gelling ingredient can be added or the gel may be formed first and then blended into the other ingredients.

Soups, Sauces, Gravies, and Salad Dressings

The main uses of high-fiber ingredients in the category of soups, sauces, and gravies are for thickening and/or to suspend particulates such as spices in these foods. Starches are the most common thickening agents for soups, sauces, and gravies, while hydrocolloid gums are used more often in dressings. The functionality of starches and gums in these applications can be found elsewhere (18; see also the Eagan Press Handbook on hydrocolloids, which is in preparation). Water-soluble fibers can be used to replace fat, add mouthfeel, increase consistency, and increase the viscosity of these product types. The ability of high-fiber ingredients to hold water aids in forming stable products that do not exhibit syneresis. Insoluble fiber types such as cellulose have the ability to hold both water and oil (see Chapter 2) and can be used in these products to aid their stability. The fibrous nature of high-fiber ingredients can also aid in providing textural properties such as increased consistency or pulpiness in tomato sauces.

Isoelectric point—The pH level at which a protein precipitates out of solution. At this level, the number of positive charges on the protein is equal to the number of negative charges.

Experimentation with fiber type and particle size can help in formulating a product with optimal mouthfeel, viscosity, and emulsifying properties.

Troubleshooting

JAMS, JELLIES, PRESERVES		
Symptom	**Causes**	**Changes to Make**
Thin consistency or lacks structure	Low gel strength	If high-methoxy pectin is used, change to low-methoxy pectin. If low-methoxy pectin is used, check pH, and/or add more pectin or calcium if necessary.
Texture too hard and/or brittle structure	Gel strength too high	If low-methoxy pectin is used, check pH and/or decrease pectin or calcium levels if necessary
Low body	Low solids; low thickening agent	Add gums (locust bean, carrageenan, or gellan).

ICINGS, FROSTINGS, GLAZES		
Symptom	**Causes**	**Changes to Make**
Cracking; formation of a hard shell	Dehydration or moisture migration	Add a hygroscopic agent such as water-soluble fiber (e.g., inulin, gum arabic). Check water activity of product and frosting to ensure that they are equal.
Too little adhesion	Excessive moisture	Check liquid levels in formulation. Add water-binding agents such as gums. Allow product to completely cool before finishing.
Icing sticks to wrapper or packaging	Too hygroscopic	Increase sucrose level. Decrease water-binding agents such as water-soluble fibers.
	Product not completely cooled	Allow product to completely cool before finishing.
Too soft	Excessive moisture	Check liquid levels in formulation. Add water-binding agents such as water-soluble fiber.

CONFECTIONERY		
Symptom	**Causes**	**Changes to Make**
Gritty texture	Presence of high-fiber ingredient	Decrease particle size of high-fiber ingredient. Experiment with high-fiber ingredient types.
Product too soft or too sticky (gummed confections)	Moisture content too high	Check processing conditions. Increase gelling agent or solids.
Product too stiff or hard	Moisture content too low or water too tightly bound	Decrease gelling agent or solids content. Increase liquid content.

MEAT, POULTRY, SEAFOOD		
Symptom	**Causes**	**Changes to Make**
Dry, crumbly texture	Moisture content low; poor water-binding ability of formula	Add or increase high-fiber ingredient(s).
	Poor adhesion of protein molecules	Add or increase high-fiber ingredient(s).
Rubbery texture	Level of binding between ingredients too high, resulting in poor release and bite characteristics	Decrease high-fiber ingredient level. Experiment with type of high-fiber ingredient.

SOUPS, SAUCES, GRAVIES		
Symptom	**Causes**	**Changes to Make**
Thin consistency, low body	Viscosity too low	Add or increase high-fiber ingredient(s).
Syneresis	Poor water-binding properties of ingredients.	Add or increase high-fiber ingredient(s).
Thick or gummy consistency	Viscosity too high	Decrease level of high-fiber ingredient(s). Experiment with type of high-fiber ingredient.

References

1. Ward, F. 1997. Hydrocolloid systems as fat mimetics in bakery products: Icings, glazes, and fillings. Cereal Foods World 42:386-389.
2. Brucker, C. E., Uhlarik, K. S., Lampe, Jr., and Bush, J. W. 1974. Lower calorie candy. U.S. patent 3,800,045. American Home Products Corp., New York.
3. Walter, D. L., and Linscott, S. E. 1995. Composition for and method of producing a fiber fortified chewy or soft-textured confection candy. U.S. patent 5,476,678. Amway Corp., Ada, MI.
4. Sheu, S. S., Yang, R. K., and Corsello, V. 1986. Soft-textured confectionery composition containing fiber. U.S. patent 4,698232. Warner-Lambert Co., Morris Plains, NJ.
5. Gonze, M., and Van der Schueren, F. 1997. Sugar-free chocolate. Candy Ind. 162(10):42-45.
6. Edwards, W. P. 1993. Using Litesse in chocolate confectionery. Food Technol. Int., Europe. 1993:139-142.
7. Kopchik, F. M. 1995. Polydextrose in soft confections. Manuf. Confectioner 75(11):79-81.
8. Kopchik, F. M. 1990. Reduced calorie bulk ingredients: Polydextrose and polydextrose II. Manuf. Confectioner 70(11):61-63.
9. Lawless, H. T. , Tuorila, H., Jouppila, K., Virtanen, P., and Horne, J. 1996. Effects of guar gum and microcrystalline cellulose on sensory and thermal properties of a high fat model food system. J. Texture Stud. 27:493-516.
10. Zumbe, A., and Schwitzquebel, T. 1990. Process for the purification of a material rich in cocoa dietary fiber. U.S. patent 4,948,600.
11. Burg, J. S. 1998. Generating yummy gummies. Food Product Design, May, pp. 121-146.

12. Demars, L. L., and Ziegler, G. 1996. Texture and structure of gelatin/HM pectin-based gummy confections. IFT annual meeting: Book of abstracts, p. 114. Institute of Food Technologists, Chicago.

13. Anonymous. 1996. Quintessential chocolates finds gum arabic strengthens centers. Candy Ind. 161(10):42.

14. Anonymous. 1999. Beef taco filling—Opta oat fiber. Appl. Bull. R991123. Opta Food Ingredients, Bedford, MA.

15. Funami, T., and Nakao, Y. 1996. Application of curdlan to meat products. I. Effects of curdlan on the rheological properties and gelling processes of meat gels under a model system using minced pork. J. Jpn. Soc. Food Sci. Technol. 43(1):21-28.

16. Backers, T., and Noll, B. 1997. Dietary fibers for meat processing. Food Mark. Technol. 11(6):4-6,8.

17. Vosen, T. R., Rogers, R. W., Halloran, J. D., Martin, J. M., and Armstrong, T. 1993. Effects of bran on sensory, storage and compositional properties of low fat beef sloppy-joes. J. Muscle Foods 4(1):71-79.

18. Thomas, D., and Atwell, W. 1999. *Starches.* American Association of Cereal Chemists, St. Paul, MN.

Special Topics

Health and Nutrition Aspects

Through the advances in science and technology, we know a great deal more about fiber and health than we did 20 years ago. Fiber has been associated with many positive effects in relation to supporting health and preventing various diseases. Both the insoluble and soluble fiber components have been associated with these benefits. While there is general consensus regarding the nutritional benefits that fiber imparts, the general public's consumption of fiber in Western countries remains below recommended levels. In the United States, the recommended daily intake is 25–30 g of fiber a day (from both soluble and insoluble sources) (1). The American public, however, consumes about 10–15 g a day (1,2). An opportunity exists to increase fiber consumption by creating a variety of good-tasting high-fiber products for the marketplace.

In general, insoluble fibers are related to colon health through their ability to increase fecal bulking, decrease transit time of waste materials in the colon, decrease fecal pH, delay glucose absorption, and bind or dilute organic compounds that have been found to be causative agents in certain diseases associated with the colon. Insoluble fibers are not digested in the stomach or small intestine, but they may be fermented by colonic bacteria to some extent in the large intestine. They have been correlated with preventing constipation, *diverticulosis*, and hemorrhoids.

Soluble fibers, in general, affect heart health. They have been associated with the control of *cholesterol* and glucose levels in the blood through their ability to delay gastric emptying, delay glucose absorption, and decrease serum cholesterol levels. These functions help to protect against heart diseases and diabetes. Soluble fibers escape digestion in the stomach and small intestine but are rapidly fermented in the large intestine. Their role in the lowering of serum cholesterol is thought to be related to their ability to bind bile acids in the small intestine, causing them to be excreted rather than readsorbed into the liver. Since cholesterol is converted into bile acids in the liver, the binding and excretion of bile acids causes an increase in the conversion of cholesterol to bile acids, thus lowering the cholesterol pool.

Both fiber types have been found to play a role in the prevention of certain cancers. The intake of insoluble fibers has been correlated with the prevention of colon cancer. The short-chain fatty acids (e.g.,

In This Chapter

Health and Nutrition Aspects
  Cereal-Based High-Fiber Ingredients
  Plant-Derived High-Fiber Ingredients
  Other High-Fiber Ingredient Sources

Labeling, Nutrient Content, and Health Claims
  Nutrient Declaration
  Nutrient Content Claims
  Other Labeling Issues
  Health Claims

Diverticulosis—A disorder in which many abnormal pouches or sacs open off the intestine.

Cholesterol—A fat-soluble compound found in animal products that is required by humans, is produced by the body, and, if present at high levels in the blood stream, is associated with increased risk of diseases of the circulatory system.

acetate, propionate, and butyrate) that are the by-products of the fermentation of soluble fibers have been linked with proper colon function. The intake of soluble as well as insoluble fibers has been shown to protect against breast, prostate, and other cancers. The exact role that these fibers play is still not known.

Many studies have been done with high-fiber ingredients to determine their efficacy and role in the prevention of these health-related issues. The following section reviews the findings for each of the principal categories of high-fiber ingredient.

CEREAL-BASED HIGH-FIBER INGREDIENTS

Oat-based. As described in Chapter 1, oat fiber is produced from the oat hull and is very high in insoluble fiber. As such, it exhibits the insoluble fiber benefits of colon health, including laxation and the prevention of colon cancer. Oat bran, on the other hand, has been correlated with the reduction of cholesterol. Since the 1970s, there has been extensive research on the role that oat bran plays in the diet. The soluble fiber component of oat bran, β-glucan, has been associated with the cholesterol-lowering properties of oats, and in the late 1980s, it was touted as the agent responsible for cholesterol-lowering (3). Many products high in oat bran were created. This major marketing trend ended when a clinical study showed that oat bran had no significant effect on the lowering of cholesterol (4). However, more recent research on the cholesterol-lowering properties of oats and oat bran has again attributed them to β-glucan. The authors of a 1992 review (5) concluded that

> there is little doubt that the gum [β-glucan] of oats is the part of its total dietary fiber responsible for whatever plasma cholesterol-lowering properties it has.

Significant evidence of this fact has led to the recent FDA approval of a health claim involving soluble fiber (see section on health claims).

Wheat-based. As with oat fiber, wheat fiber is known to function as a laxative agent and to affect colon health by reducing the risk of colon cancer, diverticulosis, etc. The research on the impact of wheat fiber on cholesterol-lowering properties has also been reviewed (5). Wheat fiber, in the form of wheat bran, whole-wheat flour, etc., has been found to play an insignificant role in the reduction of serum cholesterol, however.

Barley-based. Because of its high content of soluble fiber (i.e., β-glucan), barley bran and barley flours, like oats, are correlated with serum-cholesterol-lowering properties. Barley bran flour, also referred to as brewer's spent grain, also decreases gastrointestinal transit time and increases fecal weight (6). Barley bran flour is composed mainly of insoluble fiber. In general, insoluble fibers, such as cellulose and wheat bran, have been shown to be ineffective in lowering cholesterol. However, barley bran flour lowered the cholesterol in persons with *hypercholesterolemia* (7). The cholesterol-lowering properties of barley bran flour may be related to the lipid portion, since defatted barley bran flour has not shown any significant impact (7).

Rye-based. Because of its high fiber content, whole-meal rye flour has been correlated with the health benefits of dietary fiber. Whole-meal rye bread is reported to contain roughly three times the amount of dietary fiber as compared with white wheat bread. In a review of consumption patterns between Denmark and Finland (high rye consumption) and the United Kingdom (high wheat consumption), stool weights were higher and mean transit time was faster in the Scandinavian countries (8).

Rice-based. Rice bran has been shown to affect both laxation and cholesterol reduction in humans and animals (9,10). Rice bran, as discussed in Chapter 1, contains from about 20–30% total dietary fiber (TDF), with about 2–3% existing as soluble dietary fiber. The laxative effect of rice bran has been attributed to the insoluble portion of the TDF. Its cholesterol-reducing properties have been correlated with the lipid portion of the rice bran; if the rice bran is defatted, it has no significant cholesterol-lowering properties (10). The lipids in rice brans are known to contain high concentrations of plant sterols such as β-sitosterol and tocotrienols. These components have been shown to be hypocholesterolemic in humans and are thought to interfere with the absorption of cholesterol (9).

Corn-based. Corn bran has positive effects on several aspects of health. Some studies have shown the ability of corn bran to absorb fecal mutagens (11). Since corn bran is composed primarily of insoluble fiber, it has been correlated with laxation, preventing diverticulosis, etc. Some studies have also shown it to reduce the cholesterol content in human subjects (12). The mechanism of cholesterol reduction is not understood, but again, the reduction may be correlated with the presence of certain compounds in the lipid portion of the corn bran.

Soy-based. Extensive recent research has involved the health benefits of soy and soy products in the diet. Many of the findings have centered on the impact of soy proteins and isoflavones and their ability to significantly decrease levels of total cholesterol, *low-density lipoprotein* (LDL) cholesterol, and triglycerides. Soy fiber has also been shown to have significant health benefits. As described in Chapter 1, there are distinct differences in the composition of the dietary fiber derived from the hull of the soybean versus that from the cotyledon. In general, soy hull fibers contain a higher proportion of cellulosic fibers, while soy cotyledon fibers contain a greater proportion of soluble fiber (about 5% greater [13]). Consequently, they have different physiological functions. The cholesterol-lowering properties of soy cotyledon fibers have been well established through several clinical studies (13,14). While there is some evidence of the cholesterol-reducing properties of soy hull fiber, the results are less consistent

Hypercholesterolemia—The presence of excess cholesterol in the blood.

Low-density lipoprotein (LDL)—Molecular complexes found in the blood that attach to cholesterol. Cholesterol bound to LDL is considered bad cholesterol because it deposits on the walls of arteries.

than for soy cotyledon fiber (13). Both soy hull and soy cotyledon fibers are effective in regulating glucose levels in diabetic patients, increasing fecal bulk, and decreasing transit time (13,14).

PLANT-DERIVED HIGH-FIBER INGREDIENTS

Cellulose and cellulose derivatives. As previously mentioned, cellulose is known to have the functions associated with the insoluble portion of fiber, such as increasing fecal bulk. It has not been strongly associated with the ability to reduce cholesterol (5). The cellulose derivatives methylcellulose, carboxymethylcellulose, and hydroxypropyl methylcellulose may have some of the health benefits of soluble fibers, but their use level in foods is quite low (<2%). However, even at low levels, they may have the ability to alter the viscosity of the gastrointestinal system, which can produce certain health benefits such as improving glucose tolerance by decreasing the rate of glucose absorption.

Gums. In general, gums are sources of soluble dietary fiber and exhibit the health benefits of such fibers, such as decreasing total serum cholesterol, LDL cholesterol, and blood triglyceride levels; preventing certain cancers; and regulating glucose metabolism. Soluble fiber sources have also been associated with prevention of heart disease and diabetes. This benefit has been linked to the ability of these water-soluble fibers to increase the viscosity of the gastrointestinal system. The most prevalent work in this area has involved the use of guar gum, pectin, and gum arabic.

Inulin and FOS. Many studies have shown a relationship between various dietary-fiber-related health benefits and the intake of inulin and fructooligosaccharides (FOS). Inulin and FOS have shown promise in prevention of colon cancer by decreasing the incidence of precancerous colon lesions (15). In addition, they have been found to stimulate calcium absorption in humans who have intakes of 8–40 g of inulin per day (16). Inulin is also unique in that it has been shown to increase the proliferation of *bifidobacteria* in the colon. These bacteria are beneficial because they inhibit the growth of harmful bacteria, reduce toxins and carcinogens, activate the immune system, synthesize vitamins, and improve mineral absorption (17,18).

Konjac flour. The consumption of Konjac flour has been effective in lowering serum cholesterol and triglyceride levels (19). It has also been shown to improve glucose tolerance in persons with diabetes. Clinical studies have shown that Konjac flour is a more effective agent than guar or pectin in the treatment of diabetes since it can produce an effect when taken in smaller quantities (20).

Resistant starch. Resistant starch intake is correlated with increased fecal bulking as well an increase in the production of short-chain fatty acids in the colon (21). In addition, these starches slowly release glucose during digestion (22). Therefore, resistant starches can be useful in foods for people with diabetes.

Bifidobacteria—Species in the genus *Bifidobacterium* that can be found in the human colon and are believed to provide several health benefits.

Sugar beet fiber. Sugar beet fiber reduces serum cholesterol levels and LDL levels, as well as increasing *high-density lipoprotein* (HDL) levels (23). This effect has been correlated with the high level of pectin that is in sugar beet fiber (about 22%). It has also been shown to decrease the rate of glucose absorption, which benefits people with diabetes (23).

Pea fiber. Because of their high content of insoluble fiber, pea fibers are associated with the insoluble fiber benefits such as laxation, fecal bulking, and prevention of diverticulosis. Pea fiber has also been found to decrease the *blood glucose response* and to be an effective agent in treating *hyperlipidemia*. The latter effect may be attributed to the presence of soluble fibers in the pea fiber ingredient.

Arabinogalactan. Arabinogalactans are considered to be prebiotic fibers in that they act as food sources for bifidobacteria. As mentioned above, these bacteria are beneficial because they inhibit the growth of harmful bacteria, reduce toxins and carcinogens, activate the immune system, synthesize vitamins, and improve mineral absorption. The use of arabinogalactans in the diet also increases the production of short-chain fatty acids in the colon.

Psyllium. Psyllium is a fiber commonly used as a bulk laxative. It contains a high proportion of soluble fiber, and studies have shown it to be effective in the treatment of hyperlipidemia (5). There have been some problems with allergic reactions to psyllium, as well as the occurrence of intestinal obstructions (5). Because of its ability to bind water at low levels, psyllium intake should be accompanied by high water intake.

Fruit-derived high-fiber ingredients. Most of the health benefits that are associated with fruit-derived fiber ingredients can be attributed to the presence of pectin. Pectin, from a variety of sources, significantly decreases the serum cholesterol levels in both humans and animals (5). The ability of fruits such as prunes to cause laxation has been attributed to their content of oligosaccharides (5,24).

OTHER HIGH-FIBER INGREDIENT SOURCES

Curdlan. Curdlan is an insoluble β-glucan. As such, it exhibits the health benefits of an insoluble fiber (laxation, fecal bulking, etc.).

Chitin/chitosan. As insoluble fibers, these ingredients also exhibit the benefits found with insoluble fibers. Chitosan has been reported to be effective in increasing HDL levels (25).

Polydextrose. Polydextrose is considered a soluble fiber but has been shown to bring about the health benefits associated with both the soluble and insoluble fibers. Studies have shown the ability of polydextrose to increase fecal bulk, reduce transit time, lower fecal pH, promote beneficial colonic bacteria, increase the production of short-chain fatty acids (particularly butyrate) in the colon, and influence glucose metabolism by decreasing the rate of glucose absorption (26).

High-density lipoprotein (HDL)—Molecular complexes found in the blood that carry cholesterol. Cholesterol bound to HDL is being transported and is considered good cholesterol.

Blood glucose response—The rise in blood sugar in response to carbohydrate in the diet.

Hyperlipidemia—A condition resulting in the presence of excess lipids (fats) in the blood.

Labeling, Nutrient Content, and Health Claims

The positive impact that dietary fibers exhibit is well recognized worldwide. As described above, many statements can be made that associate foods containing dietary fiber with the prevention of certain diseases. However, the ability to make these claims on a food label depends on the regulations set forth in the region where that food is sold. Many separate governing agencies regulate and monitor the labeling of foods. For the purpose of this text, the labeling of dietary fiber and the health claims regarding dietary fiber and food products are reviewed using the regulations for labeling in the United States.

In the United States, the nutrition labeling regulations are detailed in the 1992 Nutrition Labeling and Education Act and are regulated by the Food and Drug Administration (FDA). These regulations define the nutrient declarations that are required or allowed on food labels as well the nutrient content claims and health claims that are allowed in the United States. They are found in the *U.S. Code of Federal Regulations* under Title 21. As these regulations may change and the country or region where the food is marketed may have different regulations, it is recommended that one check with the local governing agency before labeling foods.

NUTRIENT DECLARATION

The declaration of nutrients on the nutrition label is either mandatory or voluntary depending upon the nutrient. Labeling of dietary fiber is mandatory, as a subcomponent of total carbohydrate (Fig. 6-1). Labeling the soluble and insoluble components of the TDF is voluntary, but if there is a health claim regarding a component of dietary fiber, the component (i.e., soluble fiber or insoluble fiber) must be labeled as well. No official definition for dietary fiber is listed by the FDA in the *Federal Register*; however, the content of dietary fiber should be determined by the approved methods of the AOAC (Association of Official Analytical Chemists) International.

The declaration of calorie content is related to the amount of TDF in a food. The insoluble fiber content of the food is considered to contribute zero calories. The soluble fiber portion is considered to contribute to the caloric value of the food, although the actual calorie contribution can vary. For labeling purposes, the soluble fiber portion is considered to contribute 4 cal/g of food. Therefore, the insoluble portion can be (but is not required to be) subtracted from the total carbohydrate portion of the food and the remaining grams of carbohydrate then multiplied by four. Addition of insoluble fiber is, therefore, a means for reducing the calorie content of foods. In addition, caloric data for specific food ingredients is also allowed. For example, polydextrose,

Nutrition Facts

Serving Size 1 slice (31g)
Servings per package 22

Amount Per Serving	
Calories 60	Calories From Fat 9

	% Daily Values*
Total Fat 1g	2%
Saturated Fat 0g	0%
Cholesterol 0mg	0%
Sodium 90mg	4%
Total Carbohydrates 13g	4%
Dietary Fiber 5g	20%
Sugars 1g	
Protein 2g	

Vitamin A	0%	Vitamin C	0%
Calcium	6%	Iron	6%
Thiamin	10%	Riboflavin	10%
Niacin	10%	Vitamin B6	10%
Folate	10%	Vitamin B12	15%
Zinc	15%	Magnesium	10%

*percent daily values are based on a 2,000 calorie diet. Your daily values may be higher or lower depending on your calorie needs.

Fig. 6-1. Typical nutrition label for fiber-containing bread.

while it is considered a soluble fiber, is considered to contribute 1 cal/g to a food product.

NUTRIENT CONTENT CLAIMS

Foods that contain dietary fiber in significant amounts are allowed to be labeled as such according to the following guidelines as stated by the *Code of Federal Regulations* (21 CFR Part 101.54). Nutrient content claims are based on a reference amount of the food. Reference amounts vary depending on the food and are listed in the *Code of Federal Regulations* (21 CFR Part 101). The daily reference value (DRV) is equal to 25 g of TDF for an adult. If the food is not low in fat, the level of fat must be disclosed in the statement referring to the fiber content claim. See 21 CFR 101.54 for more details.

The following terms have specific definitions.

- *Good source.* The term may be used for foods that contain 10–19% of the DRV per reference amount of the food.
- *High.* The term may be used for foods that contain greater than 20% of the DRV per reference amount of the food.
- *More.* The term may be used for a food that contains more fiber than another reference food if it contains 10% more per reference amount for that food. The percentage of the amount relative to the DRV as well as the identity of the other reference food must be stated. An example claim is as follows: "contains 10% more of the Daily Value for fiber than white bread." See 21 CFR 101.54 for more details.

OTHER LABELING ISSUES

In the United States, food additives are regulated by provisions of the 1958 Food Additives Amendment to the 1938 Food, Drug and Cosmetic Act. This amendment requires that the additives used in foods must go through an approval process before use. Two types of additives are exempt from the food additive approval process. The first type consists of those that are considered "prior sanctioned" and were accepted as safe prior to the 1958 amendment. There is no complete, official listing of all prior-sanctioned ingredients, but some are listed in 21 CFR 181. The second type consists of those described as generally recognized as safe (GRAS). GRAS food additives are those that experts qualified by scientific training and experience have determined to be safe, based on either scientific procedures or common and safe use in food. Again, there is no complete, official listing of all GRAS substances, but some are listed in 21 CFR 182 and 184. The supplier or manufacturer of a high-fiber ingredient should provide adequate guidance on the regulatory status of its ingredient.

The use of materials such as food additives, prior-sanctioned ingredients, and GRAS substances is regulated as part of the regulation for standardized foods (i.e., foods that have a standard of identity) such as ice cream and cheese, as well as meat products (which are governed by the U.S. Department of Agriculture [USDA]). In some cases, warnings may need to be declared on the ingredient label. For example, polydextrose, which is approved as a food ingredient in the United States in many food applications, is known to have a laxative effect at higher levels in foods. In the United States, if a single serving of a food contains more than 15 g of polydextrose, the food label is required to bear the following statement: "Sensitive individuals may experience a laxative effect from excessive consumption of this product." Since the status of the approved levels and uses of these ingredients can change, it is best to check with the supplier of the ingredient as well as the U.S. FDA (see 21 CFR 172), the USDA (for meats), or your local governing agency for current use and labeling regulations.

HEALTH CLAIMS

In the United States, certain health claims regarding fiber and disease prevention can be made in food labeling. These claims have strict requirements, and it is best to check the latest regulation regarding the claim. Health claims are allowed only if the food product does not contain a high level of fat, saturated fat, cholesterol, or sodium (as defined by 21 CFR Sec 101.14). The health claims that are currently allowed in the United States regarding dietary fiber are discussed below. Specific details, such as the wording allowed for each of the claims, are listed in the *Federal Register*. Therefore, it is best to check the latest issue of the *Federal Register* to make sure that the information and wording for the claim are the most recent and accurate.

Claim for fiber and heart disease. *Soluble fiber from certain foods and risk of coronary heart disease—(21 CFR Sec 101.81).* This health claim relates the intake of foods low in saturated fat and cholesterol that include soluble fiber to the decreased risk of coronary heart disease. In order to qualify for the claim, the reference amount (as defined by 21 CFR part 101) of the food must contain

- at least 0.75 g of soluble fiber derived from oats (oat bran, rolled oats, or whole oat flour)
  or
- at least 1.7 g of soluble fiber derived from psyllium seed husk.

Claim for ingredients and cancer. *Fiber-containing grain products, fruits, and vegetables and cancer—(21 CFR Sec 101.76).* This health claim relates the intake of dietary fiber from the listed foods with their ability to prevent cancer. This health claim is limited to grain products, fruits, and vegetables that at least meet the "good source" nutrient content claim for dietary fiber (see above) without fortification. The food must also meet the requirements for being low fat and contain a grain product, fruit, or vegetable.

Claim for ingredients and heart disease. *Fruits, vegetables, and grain products that contain fiber, particularly soluble fiber, and risk of coronary heart disease—(21 CFR Sec 101.77).* This health claim relates the intake of dietary fiber (with a stipulation of the amount of soluble fiber) from foods such as grain products, fruits, and vegetables to the prevention of coronary heart disease. The food must meet the requirements for low saturated fat, low cholesterol, and low fat. In addition, the food must contain, without fortification, at least 0.6 g of soluble fiber per reference amount of the food. The claim does not specify an amount for the TDF in the food.

There are no approved claims for foods or dietary supplements regarding a direct relationship between dietary fiber and cancer or dietary fiber and cardiovascular disease.

References

1. Marlett, J. A., and Slavin, J. 1997. Position of the American Dietetic Association: Health implications of dietary fiber. J. Am. Diet. Assoc. 97:1157-1159.
2. Anonymous. 1996. Fiber: Why you may need more, and good ways to get it. Mayo Clinic Health Letter 14(8):4-6.
3. Horwich Allen, A. 1995. The fiber fracas has faded. Food Product Design 5(4):64-75.
4. Swain, J. F., Rouse, I. L., Curley, C. B., and Sacks, F. M. 1990. Comparison of the effects of oat bran and low fibre wheat on serum lipoprotein levels and blood pressure. New Engl. J. Med. 322:147-152.
5. Truswell, A. S., and Beynen, A. C. 1992. Dietary fiber and plasma lipids: Potential for prevention and treatment of hyperlipidemia. In: *Dietary Fibre—A Component of Food*. T. F. Schweizer and C. A. Edwards, Eds. International Life Sciences Institute, Springer-Verlag, London.
6. Lupton, J. R., Morin, J. L., and Clayton Robinson, M. 1993. Barley bran flour accelerates gastrointestinal transit time. J. Am. Diet. Assoc. 93:881-885.
7. Lupton, J. R., Clayton Robinson, M., and Morin, J. L. 1994. Cholesterol-lowering effect of barley bran flour and oil. J. Am. Diet. Assoc. 94:65-70.
8. Bach Knudsen, K. E., Johansen, H. N., and Glitso, V. 1997. Rye dietary fiber and fermentation in the colon. Cereal Foods World 42:690-694.
9. Saunders, R. M. 1990. The properties of rice bran as a foodstuff. Cereal Foods World 35:632-635.
10. Kahlon, T. S., Chow, F. I., and Sayre, R. N. 1994. Cholesterol-lowering properties of rice bran. Cereal Foods World 39:99-103.
11. Takeuchi, M., Hara, M., Inoue, T., and Kada, T. 1988. Adsorption of mutagens by refined corn bran. Mutat. Res. 204:263-268.
12. Burge, R. M., and Duensing, W. J. 1989. Processing and dietary fiber ingredient applications of corn bran. Cereal Foods World 34:535-538.
13. Lo, G. S. 1989. Nutritional and physical properties of dietary fiber from soybeans. Cereal Foods World 34:530-534.
14. Slavin, J. 1991. Nutritional benefits of soy protein and soy fiber. J. Am. Diet. Assoc. 91:816-820.
15. Anonymous. 2000. Nutritional properties of inulin and oligofructose. Tech. bull., pp. 24-26. Orafti Active Food Ingredients, Inc., Tienen, Belgium.
16. Anonymous. 1998. Improvement of calcium absorption. Company document A8-10*02/98. Orafti Food Ingredients, Inc., Tienen, Belgium.
17. Anonymous. Fruitafit—Inulin: A natural carbohydrate from chicory root. Tech. brochure. Imperial Sensus, Sugar Land, TX.
18. Niness, K. 1999. Inulin and oligofructose: What are they? J. Nutr. Suppl.:1402S-1406S.

19. Anonymous. 1994. Hyperlipidaemia—A clinical overview. In: Glucom-manan in Perspective: The Ultra-High Molecular Weight Polysaccharide for Lipid Lowering. Scientific Communications International, Ltd., Hong Kong.

20. Anonymous. 1994. Polysaccharide gels: Clinical overview. In: Glucom-manan in Perspective: The Ultra-High Molecular Weight Polysaccharide for Effective Glycaemic Control. Scientific Communications International, Ltd., Hong Kong.

21. Yue, P., and Waring S. 1998. Resistant starch in food applications. Cereal Foods World 43:690-695.

22. Anonymous. 1999. CrystaLean: Proven results in foods for diabetics. Opta Facts 12(3):3. Opta Food Ingredients, Bedford, MA.

23. Anonymous. 1994. Fibrex: The functional fiber—General product informa-tion. Tech. Brochure. Dansico, Malmö, Sweden.

24. Anonymous. 1998. Prune's role in a balanced and health-promoting diet: Carbohydrates and dietary fiber. Tech. Brochure. California Prune Board, Pleasanton, CA.

25. Anonymous. 1998. Dietary fiber and oligosaccharides. Prepared Foods 167(12):43-45.

26. Craig, S. A. S, Holden, J. F., Troup, J. P., Auerbach, M. H., and Frier, H. I. 1998. Polydextrose as soluble fiber: Physiological and analytical aspects. Cereal Foods World 43:370-375.

Glossary

Air classification—Separation of components in a solid mixture by using air.

Amorphous state—Having no crystalline state.

Bifidobacteria—Species in the genus *Bifidobacterium* that can be found in the human colon and are believed to provide several health benefits.

Blood glucose response—The rise in blood sugar in response to carbohydrate in the diet.

Bulk density—The mass per unit volume of a substance.

Cation exchange capacity—The ability to bind positively charged materials to fiber components.

Cation-exchanger—A polymer with the ability to selectively bind and release charged molecules (minerals, monomers, and polymers) under different conditions of acidity or salt concentration.

Cations—Positively charged ions.

Cellulase—An enzyme that specifically cleaves glucose units from cellulose.

Cholesterol—A fat-soluble compound found in animal products that is required by humans, is produced by the body, and, if present at high levels in the blood stream, is associated with increased risk of diseases of the circulatory system.

Colloidal dispersion—The suspension of large molecules, such as polymers, in a solution.

Conditioning (also called tempering)—The addition of moisture to the kernel.

Creaming—The process of incorporating air into a fat matrix by rapidly mixing the fat with a crystalline sugar.

Deacylation—Removal of the acetyl group from a molecule. In the case of the chitosan polymer, this increases the solubility.

Degree of polymerization—The molecular size of a polymer, e.g., the number of linked units in a starch chain.

Dilatant fluids—Fluids that increase in viscosity with increasing shear rate.

Diverticulosis—A disorder in which many abnormal pouches or sacs open off the intestine.

Dough strengthener—Material (e.g., sodium stearyl lactylate or ethoxylated monoglycerides) added to bread dough to increase the ability of the gluten to retain gas during proofing and baking.

Esterification—The reaction of a carboxylic acid with an alcohol in the presence of an inorganic acid (e.g., sulfuric acid) to form an ester.

Extraction rate—In the context of milling, the percentage of the intact grain recovered as flour.

Freeze-thaw stability—The ability of a substance to maintain its characteristics through cycles of alternate freezing and thawing.

Gelatinization—A process involving water and heat during which amylose and amylopectin become hydrated and the starch granule swells, leaching out the amylose and amylopectin.

High-density lipoprotein (HDL)—Molecular complexes found in the blood that carry cholesterol. Cholesterol bound to HDL is being transported and is considered good cholesterol.

Hydrophobic—"Water-hating" or nonpolar.

Hygroscopicity—The ability to attract and retain moisture.

Hypercholesterolemia—The presence of excess cholesterol in the blood.

Hyperlipidemia—A condition resulting in the presence of excess lipids (fats) in the blood.

Insoluble fiber—Dietary fibers that are insoluble in aqueous systems of enzymes designed to simulate the human digestive system.

Isoelectric point—The pH level at which a protein precipitates out of solution. At this level, the number of positive charges on the protein is equal to the number of negative charges.

Low-density lipoprotein (LDL)—Molecular complexes found in the blood that attach to cholesterol. Cholesterol bound to LDL is considered bad cholesterol because it deposits on the walls of arteries.

Lubricity—A desirable slippery sensation in the mouth imparted by fats.

Maillard browning—A series of reactions in foods, dependent on time and temperature, leading to the formation of certain end products, including brown pigments.

Microfibrils—Microscopic filamentous fibers.

Molding—In baking, the step in which the dough is formed into the desired shape.

Monosaccharide—A carbohydrate containing one sugar unit, usually composed of five or six carbon atoms in a ring.

Newtonian fluid—A fluid for which the viscosity remains constant at any shear rate.

Parboiled rice—Rice that has been steeped, steamed, and dried.

Polymer—A large molecule composed of monomer (i.e., single-unit) components.

Polymerize—Repeated linking of single units (monomers) of various chemical compounds, resulting in the creation of a polymer.

Polysaccharide—A carbohydrate containing several hundred, thousand, or hundred thousand sugar units (from the Greek *poly*, meaning "many").

Proofing—A step in preparing yeast-leavened products in which the dough is warmed and allowed to rise. It takes place after an initial fermentation and before baking.

Pseudoplastic fluids—Fluids that decrease in viscosity with increasing shear rate.

Resistant starch—Starch resistant to enzyme attack in the human small intestine.

Retrogradation—The process by which amylose and amylopectin polymers reassociate with each other and themselves.

Rheopectic—Describing a fluid that increases in viscosity with time.

Shear rate—The speed at which a force, such as stirring, is applied.

Shear stress—The amount of a force, such as stirring, applied to a material.

Shear—The deformation in which two adjacent planes move in a given direction while remaining parallel to each other. For instance, mixing results in shear.

Soluble fiber—Dietary fibers that are soluble in aqueous systems of enzymes designed to simulate the human digestive system.

Sponge—In breadmaking, a mixture of water, yeast, yeast food, and part of the flour, which is mixed separately in order to combine these ingredients without forming the gluten matrix.

Standard of identity—A legal standard, maintained by the FDA, that defines a food's minimum quality, required and permitted ingredients, and processing requirements, if any. Applies to a limited number of staple foods.

Syneresis—The separation of liquid from a gel; weeping.

Thixotropic—Describing a fluid that decreases in viscosity with time.

Total dietary fiber (TDF)—The total amount of dietary fiber, soluble and insoluble, in a food system.

Water-binding capacity—The amount of water a (gel) system retains after it has been subjected to a stress (e.g., centrifugation).

Water-holding capacity—The amount of water a (gel) system retains within its structure without subjection to any given addition of pressure or stress.

Yield stress or yield value—The stress that a plastic fluid withstands before it begins to flow.

Index